Manual of
Neonatal Emergency X-ray

D1628612

Manual of
Neonatal Emergency X-ray Interpretation

PWD Meerstadt

Consultant Paediatrician, Greenwich, London, UK
Honorary Lecturer, Centre for Childhood Studies (Established 1995),
Greenwich University, London, UK

Catherine Gyll

Paediatric Radiographer, Brighton, UK

WB Saunders Company Ltd
London   Philadelphia   Toronto   Sydney   Tokyo

W.B. Saunders Company Ltd   24–28 Oval Road
London NW1 7DX

The Curtis Center
Independence Square West
Philadelphia, PA 19106–3399, USA

Harcourt Brace & Company
55 Horner Avenue
Toronto, Ontario M8Z 4X6, Canada

Harcourt Brace & Company, Australia
30–52 Smidmore Street
Marrickville, NSW 2204, Australia

Harcourt Brace & Company, Japan
Ichibancho Central Building, 22–1 Ichibancho
Chiyoda-ku, Tokyo 102, Japan

A catalogue record for this book is available from the British Library

ISBN 0–7020–1567–9

Typeset by Columns Design & Production Services Ltd, Reading
Printed and bound in Great Britain by The University Press, Cambridge

Contents

Foreword

The learning curve for neonatal care is steep and frequently addressed outside the
typical working day. Investigation of infants receiving intensive care usually
involves radiography and thus the accurate interpretation of the plain radiograph
is one of the skills junior doctors must rapidly acquire. Important steps towards
such mastery include the diagnosis of normality and recognition of artefacts for
what they are, before their presence encourages an unnecessary change in
management. This manual of neonatal emergency x-ray interpretation not only
provides a fine display of the likely disorders to be seen on an intensive care unit
but, importantly, in each section builds up in easy stages from the normal to the
abnormal and clearly divides the latter according to their clinical relevance. The
manual would be a useful addition to any Neonatal Intensive Care Unit's library
as a teaching aid not only for junior doctors but also nurses undergoing specialist
training.

ANNE GREENOUGH
Professor of Clinical Respiratory Physiology
King's College School of Medicine and Dentistry
London, UK

Preface

Junior hospital doctors starting work in a neonatal unit frequently find themselves trying to interpret radiographs of a sick neonate in their care. During the day interpretation is aided by more senior members of the neonatal team and perhaps by a radiologist with neonatal experience. However, most neonatal x-rays are taken as an emergency procedure outside normal office working hours, when help may not be immediately or readily available. It is for such a situation that this manual will be a useful comparative illustrated reference. Also *each section of this manual is intended to be a structured learning package which will assist the junior hospital doctor in acquiring rapidly the basic skills of interpretation of radiographs of natural disease or iatrogenic pathology*. Such skills are a prerequisite to making rational decisions about immediate management, which often involves invasive intervention measures (e.g. intubation, insertion of chest drains) essential for the survival of the sick neonate.

It is hoped the book will also be of value to radiologists and radiographers who have limited experience of working in the field of neonatal intensive care. Radiographs are useful only if they are of high quality: radiographic skill is vitally important. Swischuk (1979) calls the neonatal radiograph 'the right arm of the clinician'; therefore some basic technical guidance is included.

In view of the aim and intended readership, *this is not a textbook of neonatal imaging and does not include references or imaging methods other than plain radiography*. Its place is as a user-friendly reference book for neonatal units and radiology departments.

We invite those who have neonatal radiographs that are better teaching examples than those included here to share these with us for a possible future edition of this manual.

Acknowledgements

We wish to acknowledge Westminster Children's Hospital (closed 1993) and Mr J. Lawson as the source of most of the radiographs, and to thank Dr F. Starer, Consultant Radiologist, Mr J. Lawson, Consultant Paediatric Surgeon, and Dr Anna Thornton, Consultant Radiologist, for their valuable comments on the text. Dr Starer, in particular, devoted considerable time to checking the radiological interpretation of the radiographs. We also wish to thank Mrs Margaret Macdonald, Publisher at W.B. Saunders, for her patience and support, without which this manual would not have been completed, Kate Bispham for typing the manuscript, and Carol Parr in the Production Department.

Introduction

The full term fetus is well adapted for the transition to extrauterine life. However the premature fetus is anatomically, physiologically and biochemically immature. Following birth, such infants will be subjected to the pressures of premature adaptation to extrauterine life and to the intensive invasive support measures necessary, the combination of which will cause particular problems/diseases. In addition, the infant passes from a sterile intrauterine environment to one which is teeming with microbial life. Colonization of body surfaces and gut is normal. Invasive clinical equipment, however, provides a route for nosocomial infection, against which the premature infant has less resistance.

An understanding of some basic neonatal terminology is necessary.

- Term newborn: 37–41
- Preterm newborn: less than 37   } completed weeks of gestation
- Post term newborn: more than 41
- Normal weight for gestational age: 10–90th centile
- Light for dates: less than 10th centile
- Large for dates: greater than 90th centile
- Neonatal period: birth to 28 days of life
- Infancy: birth to 365 days of life

Description of neonate	Birth weight (g)	Compatible gestational age (weeks)
Low birth weight	< 2500	< 37
	1500–2500	32–37
Very low birth weight	< 1500	< 32
	< 1000	< 28

When junior doctors first walk on to a neonatal unit, they find that it is like nothing they have experienced before in hospital practice.

▪ The patients are relatively tiny and deteriorate rapidly, requiring rapid diagnostic tools (e.g. x-ray imaging) which will determine appropriate intervention measures.

▪ The conditions are specific to the neonate:
  – congenital abnormalities
  – acquired diseases – hyaline membrane disease, necrotizing enterocolitis, etc.

▪ The management intervention measures are not only different but also are intensive, involving much high technology equipment.

X-ray imaging in the form of **plain radiography provides valuable clinical information** which is rapidly available to those caring for infants on the neonatal unit. However this information **needs to be interpreted in the context of the other clinical information available from the history, physical findings and results of laboratory investigations. Similarly, radiologists require the basic clinical information if they are to interpret neonatal x-rays correctly. In addition, the infant's exact age is relevant** (see pages 7, 152 and 154). All too often none of this information is provided, placing the radiologist in a difficult position, for example in deciding if collapse/consolidation is due to aspiration or infection (see Case Studies 9, 11 and 14), or whether a gasless abdomen is normal.

This manual is a brief illustrated introduction to the interpretation of neonatal emergency plain radiographs. It contains examples of not only the most common but also the most important neonatal clinical conditions requiring x-ray imaging. **Almost all of the radiographs have been reproduced at life size for realism.**

The manual concentrates on the neonatal chest and abdomen: each section has an introductory text which includes some basic guidance regarding the necessary radiographic techniques.

Limited information is given for certain life-threatening conditions (e.g. diaphragmatic hernia, oesophageal atresia) which present immediately post partum, needing instant diagnosis and appropriate management prior to surgical referral. Further clinical information is readily available in current neonatal textbooks.

Throughout, a structured/systematic approach is adopted to the interpretation of the neonatal radiograph as an aid to the beginner/learner and is intended to ingrain the approach in the reader. Additionally, as an aid to the beginner/learner, several examples of the same condition are included. Each film is reported under the following headings:

1. View

2. Technical comment

3. Clinical equipment

4. Radiological interpretation

5. Conclusion.

The conclusion may contain suggestions regarding immediate actions necessary as a direct consequence of the clinical information obtained from the radiological interpretation.

Films of a broad range of quality, including some of an unacceptable standard, have been chosen deliberately in order to illustrate technical points. In addition a chapter on clinical equipment and artefacts is included. Frequently **neonates are x-rayed to locate the position of invasive catheters, drains, lines or tubes, the malposition of which may cause serious iatrogenic disease**. In the environment of neonatal intensive care, with large amounts of high technology equipment in use on the sick neonate, artefacts are common and it is important to differentiate these from serious and treatable conditions/pathology.

RADIOGRAPHY

Accurate radiography of newborn infants is a highly skilled task. Ideally it should be assigned only to specially trained, experienced radiographers: unfortunately it is usually given to inexperienced junior staff. **The result is that the standard in district general hospitals can be unacceptably low. Interpretation of films is thus made even more difficult for the inexperienced clinician on his or her own out of hours.** In no other age group does correct diagnosis and treatment depend so much on the information provided in high quality films (Poznanski, 1976; Swischuk, 1979).

Sadly, many radiologists accept and report on substandard films, and paediatricians tend to have them repeated on the following day rather than complain. The skill needed to produce optimal films is easily learned but is not always adequately taught. Technical faults are all too common, as is apparent in many of the illustrations. Junior paediatricians need to be able to recognize them so that they are not misled. The most common are itemized, with causes and remedies, at the start of each section. However, high quality radiographs depend also upon adequate machinery. The size and rapid respiratory rates of the neonate necessitate a mobile x-ray machine which allows very short exposure times – ideally 0.01 seconds. Therefore **a high powered unit (300 mA) is essential**. It must also be highly manoeuvrable as the lack of clear floor space is a feature of many neonatal units.

Radiographic terminology

There are specific terms to describe the position of the infant and projection of the x-ray beam used to produce a variety of radiographic views of the chest or abdomen. If these are not understood the film can be misinterpreted.

The radiographic view obtained is dependent upon the infant's positioning AND whether the x-ray beam projection is vertical or horizontal.

The geometric principles are illustrated in the table overleaf.

INFANT'S POSITIONING	VERTICAL BEAM	HORIZONTAL BEAM
Lying on back (supine)	Anteroposterior view*	Left lateral view* – left side against cassette
	Cassette	Cassette
		(NB. Right lateral view* has right side against cassette)
Lying on front (prone)	Posteroanterior view	Right or left lateral view†
		Foam pad
Lying on side (lateral decubitus) right or left side up	Right lateral view* – right side against cassette	Anteroposterior or posteroanterior view*
	(NB. Left lateral view* has left side against cassette)	
Erect } Inverted }	**Not recommended/obsolete**. See introductory text to the section on the abdomen	

* Standard views
† Standard for anorectal malformations only

The term 'dorsal decubitus' is used when a lateral view is taken with a horizontal beam, of a neonate lying on his or her back, because the term 'supine', here correctly describing the neonate's position, infers an anteroposterior (AP) view (cf. 'supine/erect abdomen' on request forms).

General principles

Radiographic procedure should be standardized:

▪ The same speed film–screen combination and focus–film distance always used for every infant.

- Exposure factors noted for the first film of each infant, and, if satisfactory, used for all subsequent films.

- The time at which the film is taken noted on the film.

Correct radiographic exposure depends on the clinical query. Normally a lateral view of chest or abdomen needs increased exposure compared with the AP view. However, this does **not** apply in neonates because a lateral view is taken for a specific purpose in each case – usually to show free air.

- For suspected anterior pneumothorax, the horizontal beam lateral chest film needs **less** exposure so as to visualize the anterior chest wall clearly (see Figure 30b).

- For suspected bowel perforation, the horizontal beam lateral view needs **less** exposure so as to visualize the anterior abdominal wall clearly (see Figures 93 and 94).

- To show a nasogastric tube curled in a blind upper oesophagus (oesophageal atresia) the lateral film needs **considerably increased** exposure to penetrate soft tissues of the shoulders (Figure 52b), or the arms can be positioned out of the way as in Figure 53.

Correct exposure for an AP view of the chest and abdomen on the same film is achievable only with small preterm infants. Full term infants need two films, as the abdomen requires slightly more exposure than the chest. **Correct centring of the x-ray beam on the chest or abdomen avoids distorted film images.** Also it enables accurate localization of the tip of catheters/tubes, for example an AP beam centred on the chest may make the umbilical arterial catheter tip appear marginally 'lower', whereas one centred on the abdomen would make the endotracheal tube tip appear marginally 'higher' relative to the vertebral column. Therefore for both correct exposure and centring, separate films for chest and abdomen are required.

All nursing equipment is radio-opaque to some degree. As far as possible all leads, catheters, ventilator tubing, etc. should be cleared to the side so as not to overlie the chest or abdomen and obscure relevant detail in the film. The possibility of equipment lying **under** the infant (apnoea mattress, free end of nasogastric tube etc.) also needs to be checked. The infant must not be x-rayed lying under the hole in the incubator top: it casts a round shadow of lesser density over lung fields or abdominal organs which can be confusing (see Figures 41 and 124).

Neonates lose heat rapidly. The insulating layer of subcutaneous fat does not develop until 36 weeks so the preterm infant is especially vulnerable to hypothermia, which may precipitate a number of secondary problems. The cassette should be warmed and covered. The incubator flap or portholes must not be left open. Incubator temperature can drop 10°C in 4 minutes in models without a compensatory mechanism.

Comfort is important. An infant will not lie still if the cassette is hurting his or her back or the back of the head. Cassette edges need padding.

Handling of preterm infants may cause a marked drop in blood-oxygen saturation levels. Overhandling can lead to cardiorespiratory complications or cerebral haemorrhage. The common practice of a nurse holding the infant's limbs extended does not immobilize the patient or prevent rotation, and causes arching of the back. It may also upset the infant, who may start crying and struggling.

Erect films for obstruction/perforation and inverted views for suspected 'imperforate anus' are obsolete because of the amount of unnecessary handling involved: they should not be requested.

Radiation protection

The infant

▨ Careful collimation should include only the area of interest. The inclusion on a film of parts of the body not relevant to the clinical problem is criticized throughout the book (e.g. chest on a film requested for bowel obstruction). It is not always appreciated that this common practice results in a considerably increased radiation dose to the neonate. Extrasensitive organs (gonads, eyes, thyroid) are frequently subjected to primary radiation through careless collimation of the x-ray beam.

▨ Beam collimation should always be within the film's edges.

▨ In abdominal films, collimation should exclude male gonads.

▨ In films of chest and abdomen together to localize a nasojejunal tube or to confirm a tracheo-oesophageal fistula, the lower abdomen should be excluded from the x-ray field (see Figure 54).

▨ Tiny lead–rubber cut-out shields for gonads and thyroid are used in some units (e.g. Liverpool Maternity Hospital).

▨ To avoid repeat films (wrong exposure, wrong area x-rayed) the clinical query must be given on the request form.

The nurse

A nurse holding an infant for immobilization during x-ray exposure must always wear a protective lead–rubber apron. It is not possible to wear lead–rubber gloves inside an incubator; with accurate collimation, the dose to a holder's hands is negligible (Gyll and Blake, 1986). The nurses' hands or fingers should never be within the primary x-ray beam.

Bibliography

Dominguez, R. (1992) *Diagnostic Imaging of the Premature Infant*. Edinburgh: Churchill Livingstone

Gyll, C. (1985) *A Handbook of Paediatric Radiography*. Oxford: Blackwell Scientific Publications.

Gyll, C. and Blake, N. (1986) *Paediatric Diagnostic Imaging*. London: Heinemann.

Poznanski, A.K. (1976) *Practical Approaches to Paediatric Radiology*. Chicago: Year Book Medical Publishers.

Swischuk, L.E. (1979) *Radiology of the Newborn and Young Infant*, 2nd edn. Baltimore: Williams & Wilkins.

Swischuk, L.E. (1989) *Imaging of the Newborn, Infant and Young Child*. Baltimore: Williams & Wilkins.

The Chest

NEONATAL LUNGS

There are many causes of respiratory distress. The chest x-ray by itself may not always give the answer. Therefore the infant's exact age and history and the results of other investigations need to be considered all together to make a definitive diagnosis. An early chest x-ray (within the first few hours post partum) showing residual lung fluid (wet lung syndrome) can be misinterpreted as severe respiratory distress syndrome (hyaline membrane disease). A history of prolonged rupture of membranes suggests congenital lung infection; fetal distress and meconium stained liquor suggest aspiration.

In some of the radiographs shown alternative diagnoses are given, together with the clinical information necessary to differentiate between them.

Features of respiratory distress

Feature	Mild	Moderate	Severe
Tachypnoea	Present	Marked	Less marked
Nasal flaring	Present	Marked	Marked
Expiratory grunting	—	Present	Marked
Costochondral recession	—	Present	Marked
Sternal recession	—	Present	Marked
Cyanosis in air	—	Present	Marked

Causes of respiratory distress

Causes	Figures	Presenting at or soon after birth	Presenting as a complication of an existing disorder	Presenting after an asymptomatic period
Transient tachypnoea of newborn	18	✓	—	—
Meconium aspiration	13,15,16,17	✓	†	—
Respiratory distress syndrome (RDS)*	19,20,22,24a,26,28, 30ab,119	✓	—	—
Acute complications				
• Collapse	21	—	✓	—
• Pulmonary interstitial emphysema (PIE)	24b,25,27,28	—	✓	—
• Pneumothorax	21,25,27,28,30cd,33, 34,35	—	✓	—
• Pneumomediastinum	26,33	—	✓	—
• Pneumopericardium	34,35	—	✓	—
Collapse/consolidation	11–14,17,32a,56	✓	✓	—
Pneumonia	13,14,15,22,118,119	✓	✓	✓
Pneumothorax	23,29,31a–d,32b–d,125	✓	✓	✓
Congenital lobar emphysema	39	—	—	✓
Lung cyst	62	—	—	✓
Pulmonary haemorrhage	14	—	✓	—
Chronic pulmonary insufficiency of prematurity	—	—	—	✓
Wilson–Mikity syndrome	—	—	—	✓
Bronchopulmonary dysplasia	36,37,38,118	—	✓	—
Pleural effusion	41,42	—	✓	—
Cardiovascular (see cardiac section)	45,46,49,50	✓	—	✓
Laryngomalacia	—	—	✓	✓
Tracheo-oesophageal fistula	52–57	—	—	✓
Diaphragmatic hernia	58-61	✓	—	—
Potter's syndrome	—	✓	—	—
Hydrops fetalis and pleural effusion	—	✓	—	—

* RDS due to hyaline membrane disease (HMD) due to surfactant deficiency
† Meconium aspiration may complicate congenital infection

RDS (HMD)/lung infection

Fast neonatal respiratory rates and inadequate (low powered) x-ray machines used in many units will give movement blur which may obscure lung detail. The chest x-ray cannot reliably differentiate between RDS (HMD) and lung infection due in particular to group B streptococcus, therefore antibiotic cover is recommended before laboratory results become available. Reticular appearance to lung fields suggests interstitial infiltration (see Figures 19 and 20); 'ground glass' appearance indicates poorly aerated alveoli consolidated lung which suggests either RDS or lung infection (see Figures 22 and 26).

Collapse

The obstruction of an airway results in rapid collapse of the lung distal to it and emphysema of the adjacent lung. The most common causes are:

■ Malposition of the endotracheal tube:
  – in right main bronchus resulting in left lung collapse;
  – in right lower lobe bronchus resulting in collapse of the right upper lobe and left lung.

■ Secretions which frequently cause collapse of the right upper lobe but may affect any lobe/segment (meconium aspiration).

■ Compression by adjacent structures, e.g. tension pneumothorax, enlarged or abnormal viscera/vessels, or mediastinal masses.

Radiological features of lobar collapse

1. *General*

■ homogeneous opacification of affected lung field;

■ compensatory displacement of adjacent lung fissures and structures, e.g. diaphragm, heart, mediastinum.

2. *On AP view of chest*

(a) *Upper lobe*

■ apical shadow (see Figures 11, 12 and 56), and on the right the horizontal fissure is drawn upwards (see Figures 13 and 14).

(b) *Right middle lobe and left lingula*

■ results in the right (see Figure 56) or left heart border becoming invisible, and on the right the horizontal fissure is drawn downwards.

(c) *Lower lobe*

■ anterior bronchopulmonary segment collapse results in the diaphragm becoming invisible (see Figures 12 and 13);

■ the lower lobe collapses, particularly inferiorly and medially, giving lower thoracic (T6–10) paravertebral opacification which is partially masked by the overlying heart shadow on the left.

3. *On lateral view of chest*

(a) *Upper lobe* collapse results in displacement of the oblique fissure anteriorly.

(b) *Lower lobe** collapse results in displacement of the oblique fissure posteriorly.

  * Note the large volume of lung behind the diaphragm (see Figure 10) which is increased by lordotic positioning.

Air/gas leaks and bronchopulmonary dysplasia

Gas leaks may occur, commonly into the interstitium of the lung, pleural cavity or mediastinum, and less commonly into the subcutaneous tissues (see Figure 33), pericardial (see Figure 35) or peritoneal cavities. **These are probably all iatrogenic in preterm infants on ventilation,** due either to high ventilator pressures, usually giving bilateral lung disease (see Figure 25), and/or malposition of the endotracheal tube, giving unilateral lung disease (see Figure 31). Spontaneous gas leaks are a complication of meconium aspiration.

The pathology of hyaline membrane disease results in a stiff (non-compliant) and heavy lung. Thus with a complicating pneumothorax such lungs only partially collapse and tend to lie posteriorly in the thoracic cavity of the supine infant (see Figure 34). **The tip of the inserted chest drain should be located appropriately to drain the gas collection,** which is predominantly anterior if the infant is supine but may be posterior if the infant is prone.

Frequently, pulmonary interstitial emphysema (PIE) leads to radiological signs of early bronchopulmonary dysplasia (BPD), which may develop as early as 10 days. The point of transition in the radiological signs is arbitrary. In this manual the author has used the following criteria.

▓ PIE – predominantly honeycomb of gas locules trapped in the interstitium (see Figures 24b and 25);
– adjacent areas of alveolar compression collapse (see Figure 31c).

▓ Early BPD – predominantly interstitial opacification, often with short streaky irregular linear appearance but may be nodular due to cellular infiltration (see Figure 37).

▓ The radiological signs of late BPD (see Figure 38) include:

– interstitial fibrosis distorting regular bronchoalveolar architecture.

– adjacent areas of alveolar collapse with line shadows (linear atelectasis) and emphysema.

Technical notes

Standard view: anteroposterior (AP) with infant supine

Suggested immobilization aids (Figure 1):

▓ Cotton-wool roll under neck (especially for the preterm infant because of greater occipitofrontal diameter) to extend neck and clear mandible from upper lung fields (see Figure 14).

▓ Rolled towel nappy under legs.

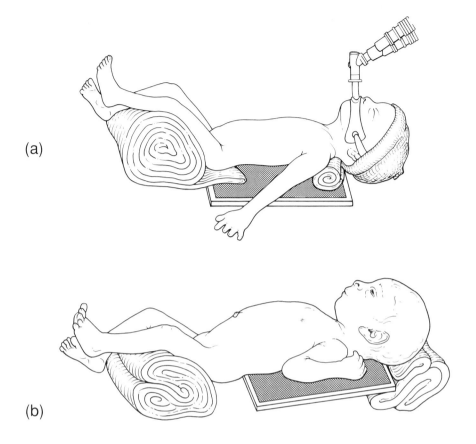

(a)

(b)

Figure 1. *Immobilization of (a) preterm and (b) full term infants. Head should be held straight*

Three common faults produce misleading appearances

1. *Expiration*

▨ Appearances: 7 or less posterior rib ends visible above right diaphragm (8 is part inspiration but is generally acceptable; 9 is optimal; greater than 10 is overinflation).
– Alters heart shape $\Big\}$ see Figure 9.
– Lung detail not seen

▨ Cause: mistiming of exposure.

▨ Remedy:

(a) exposure coincided with maximum abdominal distension (note that breathing is diaphragmatic in infancy);
(b) if on ventilator, coincided with needle swing to inspiration.

2. *Rotation*

- Appearances: anterior rib ends longer on one side than the other and posterior ribs longer on the side to which rotation occurs. **Note that symmetry of position of ends of clavicles is NOT a good index of rotation** (see Figures 5 and 121).
  – Alters heart size and shape (see Figures 47, 49 and 54).
  – Distorts mediastinal appearance especially thymus.
  – Effects a difference in translucency between lungs (see Figure 7).

- Cause: leaving infant's head lying on one side (lateral skull position).

- Remedy:

(a) head must be held or propped facing forwards (***Note:*** **the position of the endotracheal tube tip may be altered by the position of the head; therefore, because infants on ventilation are often nursed with heads turned to face the side, the ideal radiographic position may not be satisfactory for location of the tip of the endotracheal tube**);

(b) hips and shoulders must be level.

3. *Lordotic position* (as though leaning backwards)

- Appearances: straight posterior ribs, upturned upper anterior rib ends (see Figure 34).
  – Alters heart shape – apex elevated off diaphragm (see Figures 54 and 80).
  – Diaphragm masks lower lobes of lungs (see Figure 10).

- Causes:

(a) vertical x-ray beam at right angles to horizontal infant (newborn infant's protuberant abdomen causes a tendency to a lordotic view);

(b) infant's arms held extended above head, arching back;

(c) x-ray beam centred too low when abdomen included on same film, causing chest to be x-rayed with oblique (angled) ray.

(a)   (b)

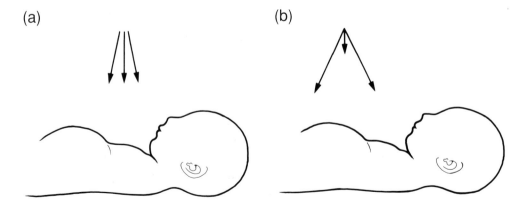

Figure 2. *(a) Correct and (b) incorrect centring for a neonatal chest x-ray.*

■ Remedy:

(a) incubator tray tilted head up 5–10°, or cassette propped head-up (see Figure 1b) or x-ray tube angled 5–10° down to feet;

(b) arms left lying by sides;

(c) if abdomen included, centring must be over chest.

Exposure should not be made when the infant is crying. Overdistended lungs are associated with pathology in babies – the same effect is produced by full inspiration when crying.

The arms should be moved out a little from infant's sides. Soft tissues of arm overlying lung can mimic pneumothorax or pleural effusion.

A sick preterm infant on a ventilator may be x-rayed prone (posteroanterior view) if that is how he or she is being nursed.

Supplementary views

Horizontal beam AP or PA view with infant lying on side

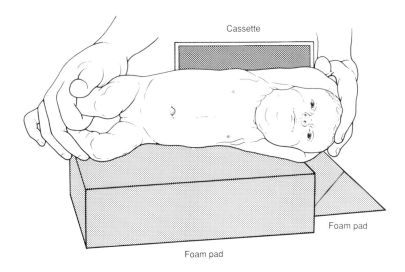

Cassette

Foam pad

Foam pad

Figure 3

To show free air or fluid in the pleural space, the infant is laid on a rectangular foam pad in the lateral decubitus position with affected side up for air, down for fluid. This view will also elucidate whether an apparent pneumothorax seen on a supine film is in fact a skinfold. The infant must be well above the level of the incubator tray: its edge produces a line artefact across the film.

Horizontal beam lateral view with infant supine

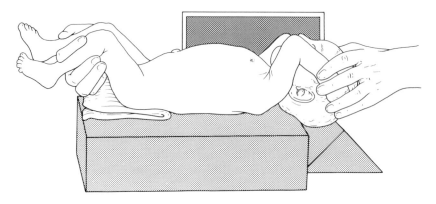

Figure 4. *Right lateral view because right side is against cassette.*

Mainly taken to demonstrate a suspected anterior pneumothorax or to check position of a chest drain. The infant lies on a foam pad as above but on his or her back (dorsal decubitus position). The arms must be held up beside the head.

Note: Exposure factors slightly less than for AP view to show anterior chest wall.

Chest and abdomen on one film: AP view supine

Chest and abdomen are included on one film for the following reasons, which mainly apply to the preterm infant:

- Localization of nasojejunal tube (NJT) or umbilical arterial catheter (UAC)/umbilical venous catheter (UVC). The insertion of a UAC cannot be confirmed reliably on a radiograph including only the upper abdomen. An initial post-insertion radiograph including the WHOLE abdomen is necessary to confirm the presence of the pelvic U-bend of the UAC.

- Congenital abnormality involving both chest and abdomen (e.g. diaphragmatic hernia, oesophageal atresia with fistula).

- First film of infant with respiratory distress because the cause may be in the abdomen (recommended by some authorities).

The x-ray beam should be centred to the chest and the infant's head shielded from primary radiation by a piece of lead–rubber on top of the incubator. Low centring (below diaphragm) increases lordotic projection of the chest. **Exposure factors are adequate also for the abdomen only in the small preterm infant. A full term infant needs increased exposure for the abdomen and two separate films should be taken**. If the request is only to localize a catheter or tube, lung detail can be sacrificed and the film exposed as for the abdomen.

CASE STUDY 1: AP VIEW OF CHEST OF TERM INFANT

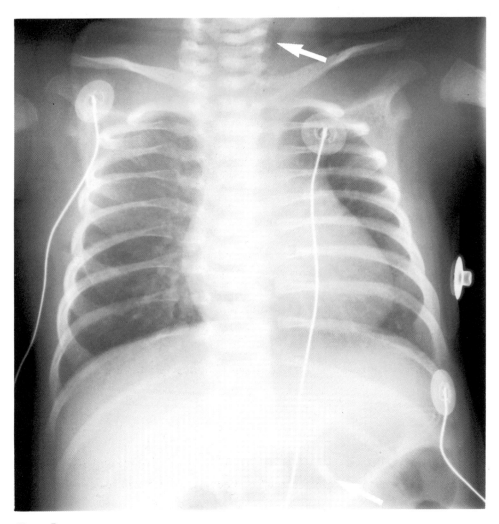

Figure 5

Technical comments

Exposure satisfactory (good lung detail visible and spine visible through heart shadow); inspiratory film (9 posterior rib ends visible above right diaphragm); rotated to the left (anterior rib ends asymmetrically placed); slightly lordotic (upper ribs almost horizontal); head facing to the left. ECG lead should have been cleared from overlying left chest.

Clinical equipment

Four ECG electrodes and nasogastric tube (NGT) in situ. Left upper chest electrode should have been moved from the field of interest.

Radiological interpretation

Trachea (arrow), mediastinum and heart rotated to the left. Mediastinum, heart and lung fields appear normal. Liver on the right. NGT tip (arrow) in stomach on the left.

Conclusion

Normal appearances of heart, lungs and upper abdomen of a term infant.

Note

- Head facing sideways usually results in rotation of the chest to the same side.
- Symmetry of position of ends of clavicles is not a good index of rotation in neonates.

CASE STUDY 2: AP VIEW OF PRETERM CHEST AND UPPER ABDOMEN

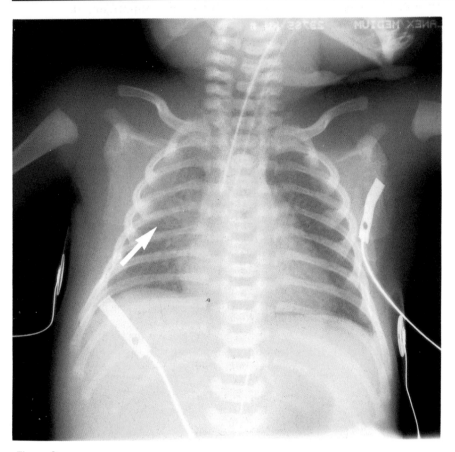

Figure 6

Technical comments

Exposure satisfactory (spine visible through heart shadow); partial inspiratory film but acceptable (8 posterior rib ends visible above right diaphragm); not rotated (anterior rib ends symmetrically placed); not lordotic (upper ribs appear to curve forwards and downwards); head facing to the left.

Clinical equipment

Four ECG electrodes, endotracheal tube (ETT) and umbilical arterial catheter (UAC) in situ.

Radiological interpretation

Mediastinum and heart normal. ETT tip at T4 which is at the level of bifurcation of the trachea. Good lung detail; no abnormalities. Horizontal fissure (arrow) seen in right lung field. UAC tip at T12.

Conclusion

Normal appearances of heart, lungs and upper abdomen in a preterm infant on intensive care.

Suggest ETT is withdrawn by 1 cm and check previous films to confirm catheter is arterial and not venous (see page 239).

Note

- Medial edge of both scapulae overlying lung fields must not be confused with a pneumothorax 'edge'.
- Slight underexposure of upper abdomen – inevitable in chest films of all but very low birth weight infants.

CASE STUDY 3: AP VIEW OF PRETERM CHEST AND UPPER ABDOMEN

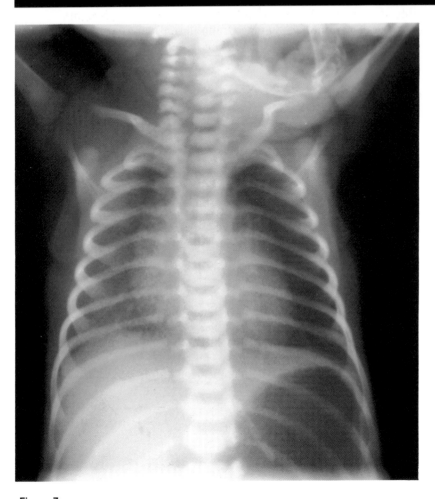

Figure 7

Technical comments

Exposure satisfactory (spine visible through heart shadow); partial inspiratory film but acceptable (8 posterior rib ends visible above the right diaphragm); rotated to the left (anterior rib ends asymmetrically placed); not lordotic (upper ribs appear to curve forwards and downwards); head facing left.

Clinical equipment

Nasogastric tube (NGT) in situ.

Radiological interpretation

Mediastinum and heart normal. Left lung field more translucent than right. No signs of a left pneumothorax. Liver on the right. NGT tip in stomach on the left.

Conclusion

Normal heart, lungs and upper abdomen. Difference in lung field translucency probably due to rotation but need to exclude a left anterior pneumothorax with a lateral view of chest with infant in the supine position and a horizontal beam projection.

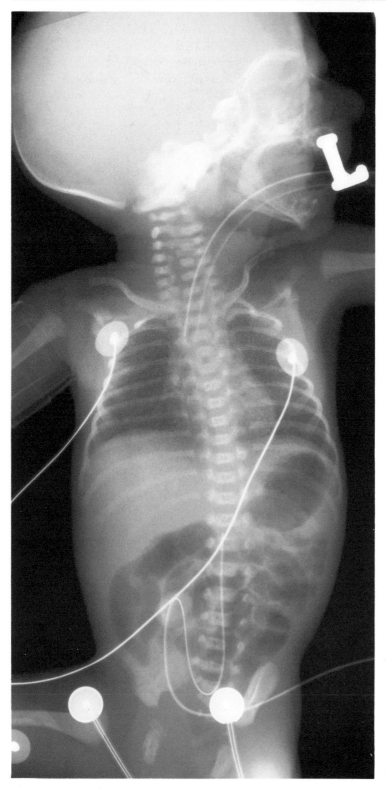

Figure 8

Technical comments

Infant's head irradiated unnecessarily (total dose increased by approximately a third). Satisfactory exposure of chest (spine visible through heart shadow) and abdomen; partial inspiration but acceptable (8 posterior rib ends visible above right diaphragm); mildly rotated to the right (anterior rib ends asymmetrically placed and posterior ribs appear longer on the right side); not lordotic (upper ribs curve forwards and downwards); head faces to the left. Left ECG lead should have been moved from field of interest.

Clinical equipment

Five skin electrodes, an endotracheal tube (ETT) and an umbilical arterial catheter (UAC) in situ. Left chest ECG electrode should have been placed on left shoulder, and left lower anterior abdominal skin probe on left lateral abdomen, away from fields of interest.

Radiological interpretation

Mediastinum and heart normal. Lung fields normal and symmetrical in translucency. Tip of ETT at T3 at carina. Abdomen – normal liver, stomach and bowel gas shadows. No evidence of bowel wall thickening or pneumatosis intestinalis suggestive of necrotizing enterocolitis. Tip of UAC at L1–2.

Conclusion

Normal heart, lungs and abdomen of a preterm infant on intensive care. ETT tip too low: suggest withdrawal by 1 cm. UAC tip at level of renal arteries: suggest withdrawal by 1cm.

Note

▪ Satisfactory exposure of chest and abdomen simultaneously is possible **only** in such very low birth weight infants.

CASE STUDY 5: AP VIEWS OF CHEST AND UPPER ABDOMEN OF PRETERM INFANT

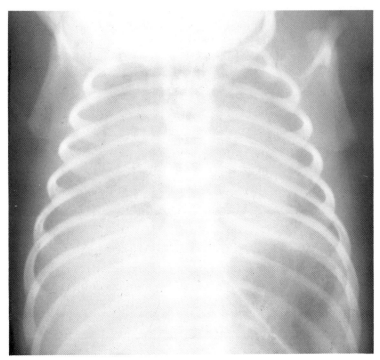

Figure 9a

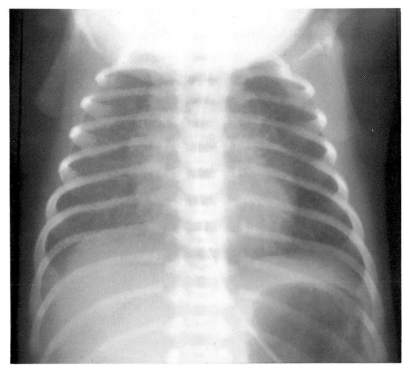

Figure 9b

Technical comments

Exposure satisfactory (spine visible through heart shadow); Figure 9a – expiratory film (7 posterior rib ends visible above the right diaphragm), Figure 9b – part inspiratory film (8 posterior rib ends visible above the right diaphragm); not rotated (anterior rib ends symmetrically placed); not lordotic (upper ribs appear to curve forwards and downwards); head facing forward.

Clinical equipment

Nasogastric tube (NGT) in situ.

Radiological interpretation

Figure 9a – Heart appears enlarged and lungs opacified – poorly aerated. Position of diaphragms unclear. Liver on the right. Stomach on the left.

Figure 9b – Widened upper mediastinum; probably large thymus. Heart not enlarged. Lung fields appear normal. Diaphragms clearly seen. Liver on the right. Stomach on the left.

NGT passing into stomach; tip off the film.

Conclusion

Normal mediastinum, heart and lungs in a preterm infant.

Note

▨ Figure 9b taken immediately after Figure 9a.

▨ Films exposed in expiration may be misleading (see page 11) and must be repeated.

CASE STUDY 6: LATERAL VIEW OF CHEST AND UPPER ABDOMEN OF TERM INFANT

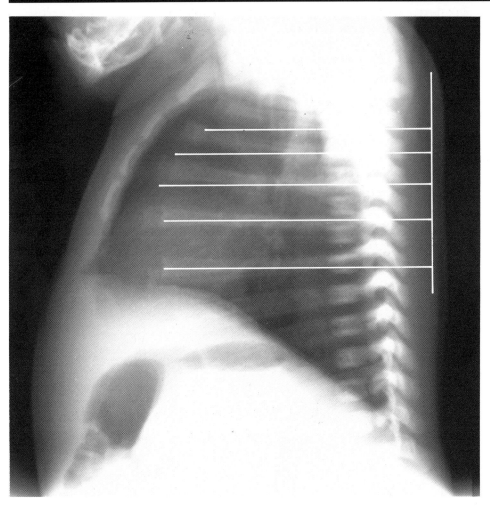

Figure 10

Technical comments

Exposure satisfactory; not significantly rotated (anterior rib end locations almost coincide); flexed neck so that on an AP view mandible would lie over lung apices; arms raised to sides of infant's head.

Clinical equipment

None.

Radiological interpretation

Raising the infant's arms places the infant's chest in a lordotic position. An AP film, as indicated by the lines drawn, would show horizontal mid-thoracic ribs and upper ribs appearing to curve forwards and upwards (Figure 15) instead of forwards and downwards.

Conclusion

Normal heart, lungs and upper abdomen.

Note

- How much of the lower lobe would lie behind the diaphragm on an AP view.
- Lordotic positioning alters the appearance of the heart (see page 12).

CASE STUDY 7: AP VIEW OF PRETERM CHEST AND UPPER ABDOMEN

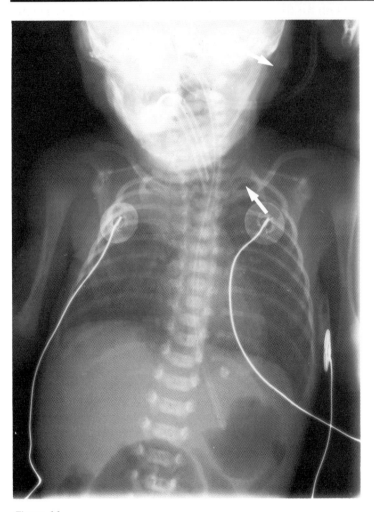

Figure 11

Technical comments

Exposure satisfactory (spine visible through heart shadow); slightly overinflated (10 posterior rib ends visible above the right diaphragm); slight rotation to the left (anterior rib ends slightly asymmetrically placed); not lordotic (upper ribs appear to curve forwards and downwards); head facing forwards. ECG leads should have been removed from the field of interest. Infant's eyes irradiated unnecessarily.

Clinical equipment

Endotracheal tube (ETT), nasogastric tube (NGT), left scalp central venous line (arrow) and three ECG electrodes in situ. ECG electrodes should be placed on shoulders and abdomen clear of lung fields.

Radiological interpretation

Mediastinum and heart shadow appear normal. ETT tip at T1–2. Right upper lobe collapse consolidation. Otherwise lung fields appear normal. Tip of central venous line (arrow) at junction of left jugular and subclavian veins. Tip of NGT in stomach. No gas under diaphragms. Normal appearance of liver, stomach and bowel gas patterns. Calcification below 11th left rib.

Conclusion

Right upper lobe collapse in a preterm infant on intensive care. Calcification is possibly adrenal.

CASE STUDY 8: AP VIEW OF PRETERM CHEST AND ABDOMEN

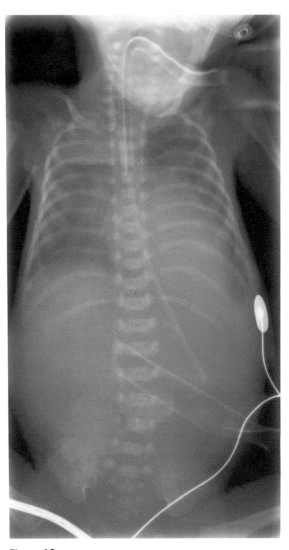

Figure 12

Technical comments

Exposure satisfactory for both chest and abdomen (see page 5); inspiratory film (9 posterior rib ends visible above the right diaphragm); not rotated (anterior rib ends symmetrically placed); not lordotic (upper ribs appear to curve forwards and downwards); head facing forwards.

Clinical equipment

ECG electrode, endotracheal tube (ETT), nasogastric tube (NGT) and left leg central venous line and abdominal dressing in situ.

Radiological interpretation

Narrow upper mediastinum. Heart shadow not enlarged. ETT tip at T4–5, i.e. at carina. Right upper lobe collapse consolidation. Left diaphragm invisible indicating left lower lobe collapse. NGT tip in abdomen. No gas in stomach or bowel. Central venous line tip at T7. Artefacts over abdomen are surgical dressing.

Conclusion

Right upper lobe collapse consolidation and left lower lobe collapse in a preterm infant on intensive care. ETT tip too low: suggest withdrawal by 1 cm.

Note

- See page 152 for causes of gasless abdomen.

CASE STUDY 9: PA VIEW OF CHEST AND ABDOMEN OF PRETERM INFANT

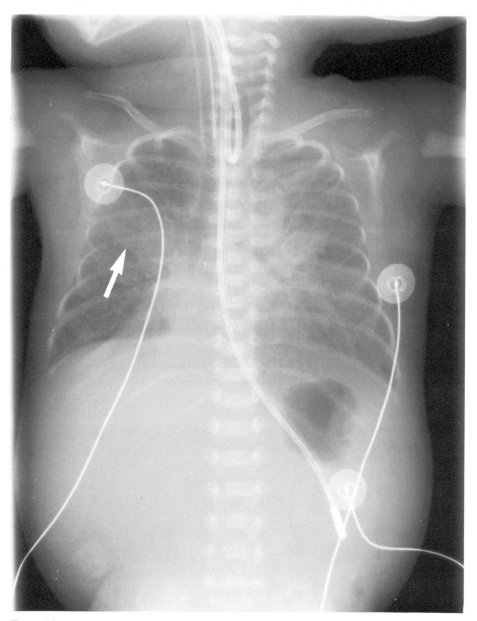

Figure 13

Technical comments

Exposure satisfactory (spine visible though heart shadow); slightly overexpanded (9–10 posterior rib ends visible above right diaphragm); slightly rotated to the right (anterior rib ends asymmetrically placed); head facing to the right. ECG leads should have been moved from field of interest. *Note:* this film was taken with infant prone.

Clinical equipment

Three ECG electrodes, endotracheal tube (ETT), nasogastric tube (NGT) and nasojejunal tube (NJT) in situ.

Radiological interpretation

Mediastinum, trachea and heart rotated to the right. ETT tip at T1–2. Rotation has made left hilum appear prominent. Bilateral, generalized opacification of lung fields with streaky appearance. Right horizontal fissure (arrow) displaced upwards and left diaphragm invisible. Right diaphragm visible. Liver on the right. NGT tip in stomach on the left. NJT doubled up in pocket of gas in oesophagus but tip in stomach. No bowel gas visible. Right iliac fossa opacity.

Conclusion

Partial right upper lobe collapse and left lower lobe collapse. Appearance of lung fields is compatible with aspiration of liquor or infection in a preterm infant on intensive care. Inspissated/calcified meconium in right iliac fossa.

Suggest doubled up loop of NJT is withdrawn and an infection screen.

Note

▧ Clinicians must give radiologist all relevant birth details, for example whether there has been prolonged rupture of membranes or fetal distress.

▧ See page 152 for causes of gasless abdomen.

CASE STUDY 10: AP VIEW OF PRETERM CHEST AND UPPER

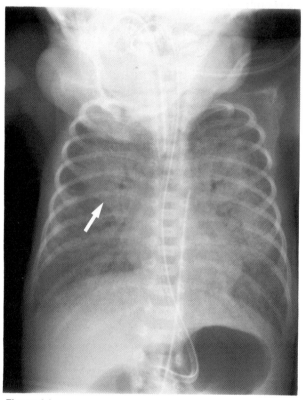

Figure 14

Technical comments

Exposure satisfactory (spine visible through heart shadow); overexpanded (10 posterior rib ends visible above right diaphragm); not rotated (anterior rib ends symmetrically placed); not lordotic (upper ribs appear to curve forwards and downwards); head facing forwards. A small roll of cotton wool under the shoulders would allow enough neck extension to clear the soft tissues of the lower face from overlying the lung apices.

Clinical equipment

Endotracheal tube (ETT), nasogastric tube (NGT) and umbilical arterial catheter (UAC) in situ.

Radiological interpretation

Mediastinum and heart shadow – normal appearance. ETT tip at T3–4. Tracheal bifurcation and air bronchogram clearly seen. Bilateral diffuse/disseminated patchy consolidation of lung fields. Horizontal fissure (arrow) appearance indicates collapse consolidation of the right upper lobe. Tip of UAC high at T6. NGT in stomach at pylorus. Flat diaphragms. Normal appearance to liver and stomach air bubble.

Conclusion

Right upper lobe collapse/consolidation and widespread consolidation compatible with an infective process in a preterm infant on intensive care. Poor aeration of lungs cannot be due to inadequate ventilation because chest overexpanded.
   Suggest UAC should be withdrawn by 2.5 cm.
   Differential diagnosis – pulmonary haemorrhage if blood in ETT.

Note

▨ Head facing forward and chin depressed – the above positional correction would alter position of tip of ETT.

CASE STUDY 11: AP VIEW OF CHEST AND ABDOMEN OF A NEARLY TERM INFANT

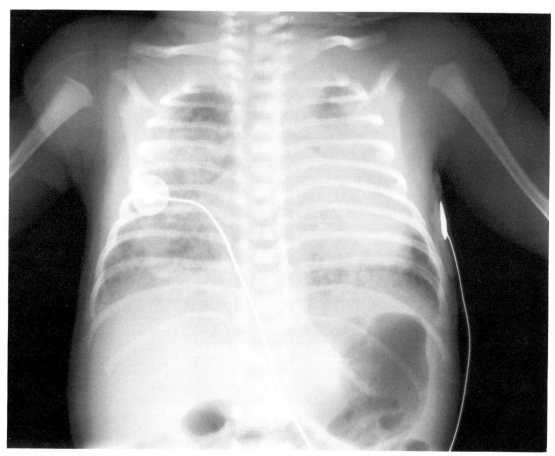

Figure 15

Technical comments

Exposure satisfactory (spine visible through heart shadow); inspiratory film (9 posterior rib ends visible above right diaphragm); slightly rotated to the left (posterior ribs appear longer on the left); markedly lordotic (upper ribs appear to curve forwards and upwards). ECG lead should have been cleared from the field of interest.

Clinical equipment

Two ECG electrodes, nasogastric tube (NGT) and right arm central venous line in situ.

ECG electrode on right chest should have been placed on right shoulder away from field of interest.

Radiological interpretation

Patchy consolidation of both lung fields. Apparent enlargement of heart but evaluation difficult on this lordotic film. Liver not enlarged. Therefore not in congestive cardiac failure. NGT tip in stomach. Liver, stomach and bowel gas shadows appear normal.

Conclusion

Patchy pneumonic changes in both lung fields due to either aspiration or infection depending on details of birth history.

Note

- Clinicians must give radiologist all relevant information, for example whether there has been prolonged rupture of membranes or meconium stained liquor.
- Distal end of central venous line could be located by injection of 1–2 ml of contrast medium (discuss with radiologist) (see Figure 117).

CASE STUDY 12: AP VIEW OF TERM CHEST AND UPPER ABDOMEN

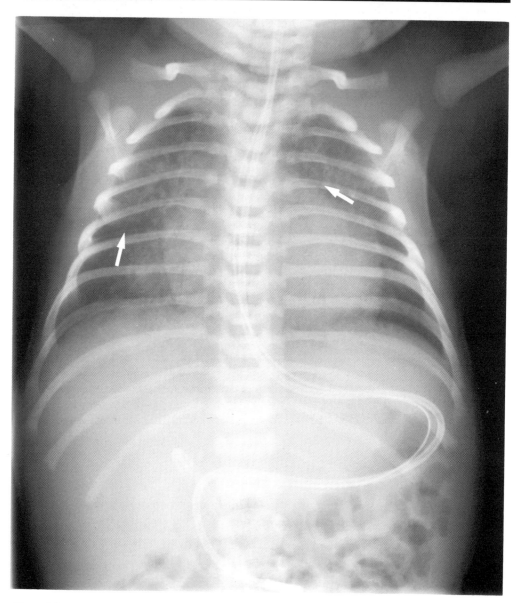

Figure 16

Technical comments

Exposure satisfactory (spine visible through heart shadow); partial inspiration but acceptable (8 posterior rib ends visible above right diaphragm); not rotated (anterior rib ends symmetrically placed); lordotic (upper ribs appear to curve forwards and upwards); head facing forwards.

Clinical equipment

Nasogastric (NGT) and nasojejunal (NJT, metal end) tubes in situ.

Radiological interpretation

Patchy consolidation of both lung fields. Fine streak of air in left mid-zone (arrow) due to pulmonary interstitial emphysema. Right lung horizontal fissure visible (arrow). No pneumothorax. No difference in translucency of lung fields. Heart shadow marginally enlarged. This could be either (1) apparent enlargement due to poor inflation, or (2) actual enlargement with some enlargement of liver. Bowel gas shadows normal. Impossible to interpret anatomical location of distal ends of catheters.

Conclusion

Patchy consolidation of both lung fields, early pulmonary interstitial emphysema and possible signs of right heart failure due to meconium aspiration (early stage) in a term infant. (Birth history of fetal distress and meconium stained liquor followed by respiratory distress.)

Note

▧ Pneumothorax is a common complication.

CASE STUDY 13: AP VIEW OF FULL TERM CHEST AND UPPER ABDOMEN

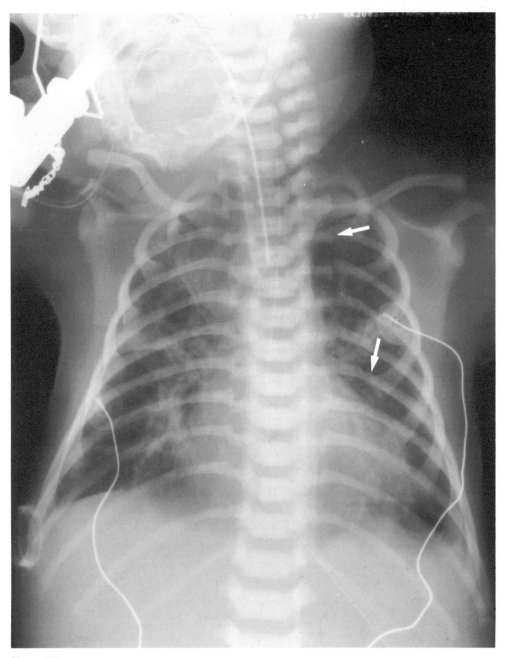

Figure 17

Technical comments

Exposure satisfactory (spine visible through heart shadow); overinflated (10 posterior rib ends visible above the right diaphragm); rotated to the right (anterior rib ends asymmetrically placed and posterior ribs appear longer on the right); not lordotic (upper ribs appear to curve forwards and downwards); head facing right for true positioning of endotracheal tube tip but has caused rotation to the right.

Clinical equipment

Two ECG electrodes, an endotracheal tube (ETT), Tunstall connector, a nasogastric tube (NGT) and a sensor base of a transcutaneous blood gas monitor in situ.

Radiological interpretation

Mediastinum and heart appear normal. ETT tip at T3. Right upper lobe collapse consolidation. Patchy consolidation in both mid-lung fields. Translucent peripheral lung fields indicative of air trapping. No evidence of a pneumothorax. Translucent streaks (arrows) suggestive of pulmonary interstitial emphysema. Diaphragms flattened. Gasless upper abdomen. NGT passing into stomach but tip off the film.

Conclusion

Right upper lobe collapse consolidation and widespread patchy consolidation in both lung fields with air trapping due to meconium aspiration (late stage) in a term infant.

Note

▓ Pneumothorax is a common complication.

CASE STUDY 14: AP VIEW OF TERM CHEST AND UPPER ABDOMEN

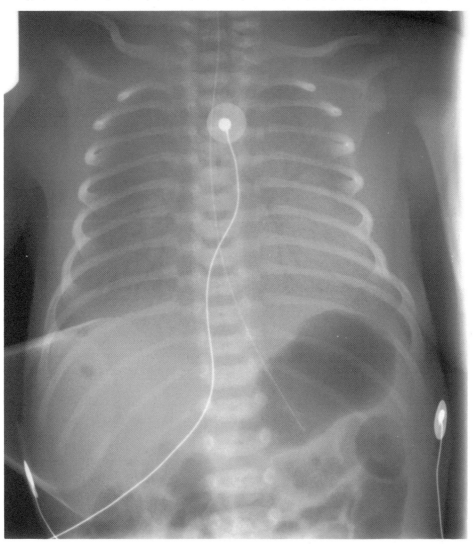

Figure 18

Technical comments

Exposure acceptable but poor contrast; inspiratory film (9 posterior rib ends visible above the right diaphragm); not rotated (anterior rib ends symmetrically placed); slightly lordotic (upper ribs horizontal). Face mask should have been removed.

Clinical equipment

Three ECG electrodes, nasogastric tube (NGT) in situ and a rubber funnel face mask underlying or overlying the right upper abdomen.

Radiological interpretation

Mediastinum and heart outline unclear. Air bronchogram seen over heart shadow with linear lung markings extending distally from hila, fluid in the horizontal fissure and slight opacification of the lung fields. Liver on the right. Stomach on the left. NGT tip in stomach. Bowel gas pattern appears normal.

Conclusion

Term newborn infant with the early appearance of delayed resorption of fetal lung fluid, as distinct from aspiration, leading to transient tachypnoea of the newborn. Later appearances show clearing of opacification of lung fields leaving residual linear lung markings extending distally from hila, and fluid in the horizontal fissure.

Note

Clinicians must give radiologist all relevant birth details, for example whether birth was by Caesarean section, or there has been prolonged rupture of membranes or meconium stained liquor.

CASE STUDY 15: AP VIEW OF PRETERM CHEST

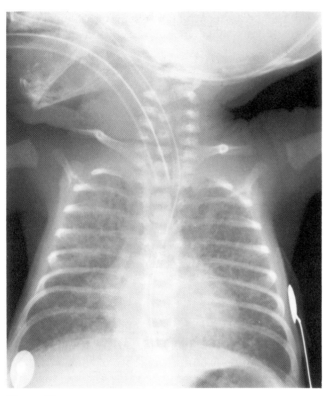

Figure 19

Technical comments

Exposure satisfactory (spine just visible through heart shadow); inspiratory film (9 posterior rib ends visible above the right diaphragm); not rotated (anterior rib ends symmetrically placed); lordotic (horizontal ribs 1–3); head facing right for true positioning of endotracheal tube tip.

Clinical equipment

Two ECG electrodes, endotracheal tube (ETT) and nasogastric tube (NGT) in situ.

Radiological interpretation

Mediastinum and heart normal. ETT tip at T1. Lung fields show generalized reticular shadowing. No evidence of pneumothorax. NGT passing into stomach. Liver on the right. Stomach on the left.

Conclusion

Reticular lung appearances compatible with the respiratory distress of early hyaline membrane disease in a markedly preterm infant on intensive care.

CASE STUDY 16: AP VIEW OF PRETERM CHEST AND UPPER ABDOMEN

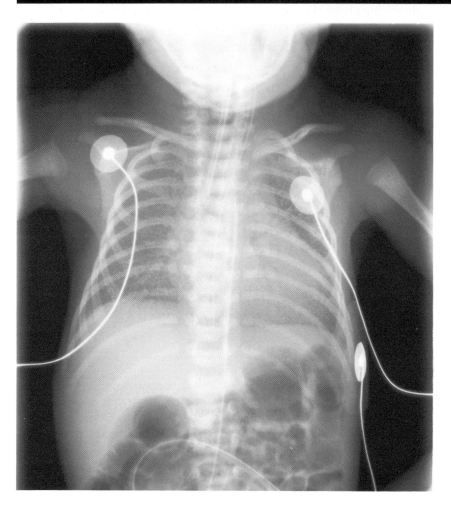

Figure 20

Technical comments

Exposure satisfactory (spine visible through heart shadow); inspiratory film (9 posterior rib ends visible above the right diaphragm); some rotation to the left (anterior rib ends asymmetrically placed and posterior ribs appear longer on the left); not lordotic (upper ribs appear to curve forwards and downwards); head facing forwards.

Clinical equipment

Three ECG electrodes, endotracheal tube (ETT), nasogastric tube (NGT) and umbilical arterial catheter (UAC) in situ. Upper left chest ECG electrode incorrectly placed overlying lung field.

Radiological interpretation

Mediastinum and heart normal. ETT tip at T4 – bifurcation of trachea. Lung fields – air bronchograms clearly visible through heart shadow and generalized reticular shadowing in both lung fields. Equal translucency of lung fields and no evidence of pneumothorax. Upper abdomen – normal liver and bowel gas shadows. NGT tip in lower oesophagus. UAC tip high at T4.

Conclusion

Lung field appearances suggestive of/compatible with respiratory distress of early hyaline membrane disease in a markedly preterm infant on intensive care.
 Suggest appropriate adjustment of ETT, NGT and UAC tip positions.

Note

▨ Initial post UAC insertion film must include whole of chest and abdomen (see pages 239 and 257).

CASE STUDY 17: AP VIEW OF PRETERM CHEST AND UPPER ABDOMEN

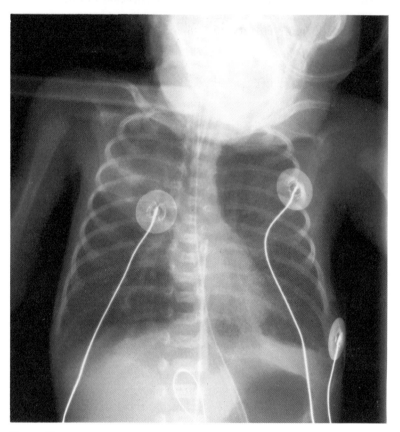

Figure 21

Technical comments

Exposure satisfactory (spine visible through heart shadow); gross overinflation (11 posterior rib ends visible above the right diaphragm); slightly rotated to the left (anterior rib ends asymmetrically placed); not lordotic (upper ribs appear to curve forwards and downwards); head facing forwards. A roll of cotton wool under the shoulders would allow enough neck extension to clear the soft tissues of the lower face from overlying the lung apices. Note that the location of the endotracheal tube tip is affected by the position of the head (see page 12).

Clinical equipment

Endotracheal tube (ETT), nasogastric tube (NGT), umbilical arterial catheter (UAC) and three ECG electrodes in situ. The ECG electrodes should have been placed on the shoulders and abdomen clear of the lung fields.

Radiological interpretation

Long thin mediastinum and heart shadow, flat diaphragms and splayed right ribs, caused by gross overinflation. ETT tip at T2–3. Air bronchogram just visible. Horizontal fissure appearance indicates collapse consolidation of the right upper lobe. Increased translucency of the right lower lung field suggests a possible small, possibly loculated pneumothorax. Reticular pattern to left lung field. Tip of UAC at T7. NGT passing into stomach but location of tip off the film. No gas under diaphragms.

Conclusion

Right upper lobe collapse consolidation, a possible small loculated pneumothorax on the right and gross overinflation in a preterm infant on intensive care. Probable respiratory distress syndrome but consider infection.
   Suggest:

1. Review of ventilator pressures.

2. An AP view of chest with infant in the left lateral decubitus position (lying on left side with right side uppermost) and a horizontal beam projection to demonstrate small right pneumothorax.

3. Withdrawal of UAC by 2 cm.

4. Infection screen.

CASE STUDY 18: AP VIEW OF PRETERM CHEST AND UPPER ABDOMEN

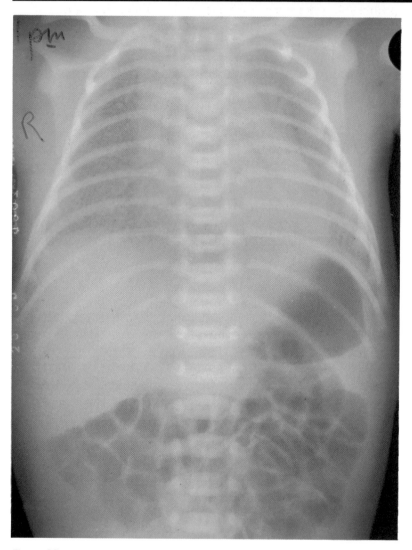

Figure 22

Technical comments

Exposure unsatisfactory: grey film – no contrast or detail (spine visible through heart shadow); inspiratory film (9 posterior rib ends visible above the right diaphragm); not rotated (anterior rib ends symmetrically placed); not lordotic (upper ribs appear to curve forwards and downwards).

Clinical equipment

Nil.

Radiological interpretation

Mediastinum and heart appear normal. Air bronchogram over heart shadow. Ground glass (homogeneous opacification) appearance to both lung fields. Liver on the right. Stomach on the left. Bowel gas shadows appear normal.

Conclusion

Lung field appearances compatible with either hyaline membrane disease or group B streptococcal pneumonia in a preterm infant.
    Suggest infection screen.

CASE STUDY 19: AP VIEW OF PRETERM CHEST AND UPPER ABDOMEN

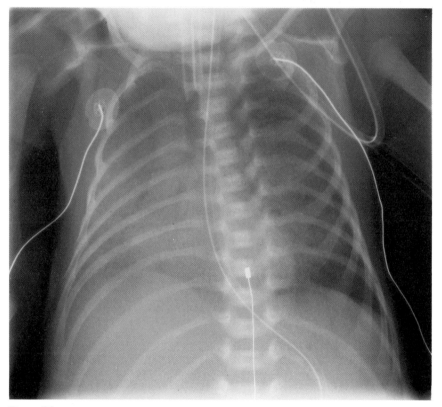

Figure 23

Technical comments

Exposure satisfactory (spine clearly visible through heart shadow); inspiratory film (9/10 posterior rib ends visible above the right diaphragm); markedly rotated to the right (anterior rib ends asymmetrically placed); not lordotic (upper rib ends appear to curve forwards and downwards); head facing forwards.

Clinical equipment

Two ECG electrodes, endotracheal tube (ETT), nasogastric tube (NGT), umbilical arterial electrode/catheter (UAC) and right arm central venous line in situ.

Radiological interpretation

Mediastinum and heart appear to be displaced because of rotation to the right. ETT tip at T2. Air in the trachea and right bronchus clearly seen over upper mediastinum and heart shadows respectively. Lung field appearances cannot be interpreted. Increased translucency of left lung field with indistinct line parallel to left mid-rib-cage caused by a combination of rotation and either a pneumothorax or a skin crease respectively. (Suggestive of skin crease if lung markings can be seen distally/externally.) NGT tip is off the film. UAC tip at T9. Central venous line tip in superior vena cava.

Conclusion

Unacceptable film: this distorted view is not diagnostic. Possible small left pneumothorax (or skin crease) in a preterm infant on intensive care.
   Suggest:

1. Repeat chest x-ray correctly positioned.

2. Supplementary AP view to rule out a pneumothorax (infant lying on the right side, left side up, and a horizontal beam projection).

CASE STUDY 20: AP VIEWS OF PRETERM CHEST AND UPPER ABDOMEN

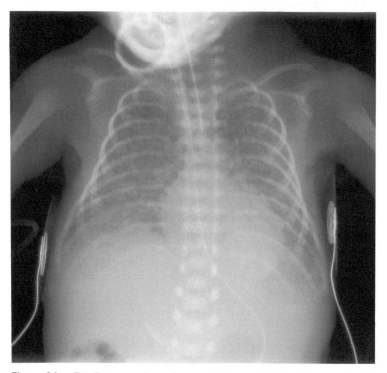

Figure 24a. *This Figure and Figure 24b are of the same infant and consecutive films.*

Technical comments

Exposures satisfactory (spine visible through heart shadow); Figure 24a overinflated (10/11 posterior rib ends visible above right diaphragm) and Figure 24b underinflated but acceptable (8 posterior rib ends visible above right diaphragm); Figure 24a not rotated and Figure 24b rotated to the left (note position of anterior rib ends and compare length of posterior ribs on each side); Figure 24a not lordotic (upper ribs appear to curve forwards and downwards) and Figure 24b lordotic (upper ribs horizontal). *Note:* these films are not comparable due to positioning faults in Figure 24b.

Clinical equipment

Endotracheal tube (ETT), nasogastric tube (NGT), two ECG electrodes and transcutaneous sensor bases in situ. The sensor bases in Figure 24b should be removed from overlying the left lung apex.

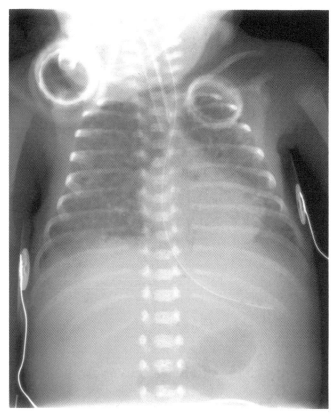

Figure 24b

Radiological interpretation

Figure 24a – Narrow upper mediastinum due to overinflation. Heart shadow appears normal. ETT tip low at T4–5, i.e. at the tracheal bifurcation. Air bronchogram just visible over the heart shadow. Reticulogranular opacification of both lung fields. Difficult to visualize diaphragms. No gas in stomach but some gas in bowel. NGT tip at pylorus.

Figure 24b – Mediastinum and heart appear displaced to the left by the rotation. ETT tip at T2–3. Air bronchogram visible over the heart shadow. Reticulogranular shadowing with translucent lacunae suggestive of early pulmonary interstitial emphysema. Little gas in abdomen. NGT tip in stomach.

Conclusion

Severe respiratory distress and early pulmonary interstitial emphysema probably due to hyaline membrane disease.

Differential diagnosis – nosocomial infection in particular group B streptococcus. Infection screen required.

CASE STUDY 21: AP VIEW OF PRETERM CHEST AND WHOLE ABDOMEN

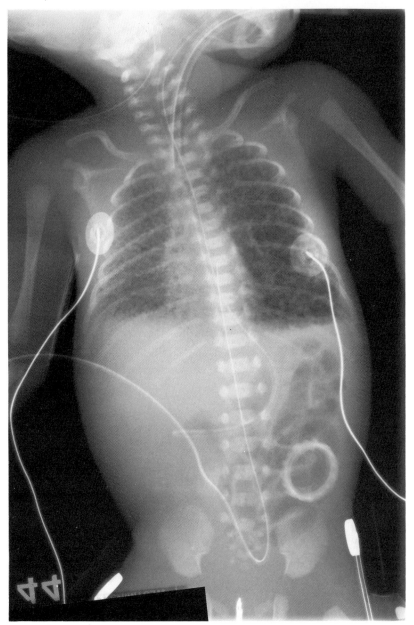

Figure 25

Technical comments

Exposure satisfactory (spine visible through heart shadow); inspiratory film (9 posterior rib ends visible above the right diaphragm); overinflation on the left (10 posterior rib ends visible above the left diaphragm); slight rotation to the right (anterior rib ends asymmetrically placed and posterior ribs appear longer on the right); not lordotic (upper ribs appear to curve forwards and downwards). Head facing to the left.

Clinical equipment

Two ECG electrodes, two skin probes, a transcutaneous sensor base, an endotracheal tube (ETT), nasogastric tube (NGT), umbilical arterial catheter (UAC) and rectal thermometer probe in situ.

Radiological interpretation

Mediastinum and heart displaced to the right. ETT tip at T2. Bilateral pulmonary interstitial emphysema with difference in translucency between right and left lung fields. Overinflation of left chest results in mediastinal/cardiac displacement, gross flattening of the left diaphragm and splaying of left rib cage. The combination of these radiological signs suggests an anterior tension pneumothorax. NGT at pylorus. Liver and bowel gas shadows appear normal. UAC tip at T7.

Conclusion

Gross pulmonary interstitial emphysema of left lung and probable left anterior tension pneumothorax in a preterm infant on intensive care.

Suggest a left lateral view of chest with infant in dorsal decubitus (supine) position with horizontal x-ray beam projection to confirm anterior pneumothorax.

CASE STUDY 22: AP VIEW OF PRETERM CHEST AND UPPER ABDOMEN

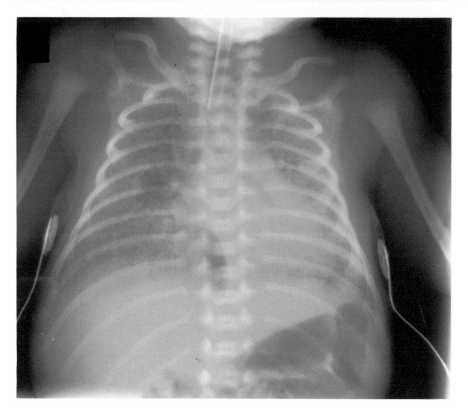

Figure 26

Technical comments

Exposure satisfactory (spine visible through heart shadow); inspiratory film (8/9 posterior rib ends visible above right diaphragm); slightly rotated to the right (anterior rib ends asymmetrically placed and posterior ribs appear longer on the right); not lordotic (upper ribs appear to curve forwards and downwards).

Clinical equipment

Two ECG electrodes and an endotracheal tube (ETT) in situ.

Radiological interpretation

Mediastinum and heart not displaced. Heart outline unclear because of lung pathology. ETT tip at T2–3. Air bronchogram clearly visible over heart shadow. Generalized increased opacification (ground glass appearance) of both lung fields with areas of translucency in right mid-lung field and along lower right mediastinal border. Diaphragms' position unclear. Liver on the right. Stomach on the left.

Conclusion

Early right lung gas leak, mediastinal gas and lung field appearances compatible with severe hyaline membrane disease in a preterm infant on intensive care.

Differential diagnosis – nosocomial infection in particular group B streptococcus. Infection screen required.

CASE STUDY 23: AP VIEW OF PRETERM CHEST AND UPPER ABDOMEN

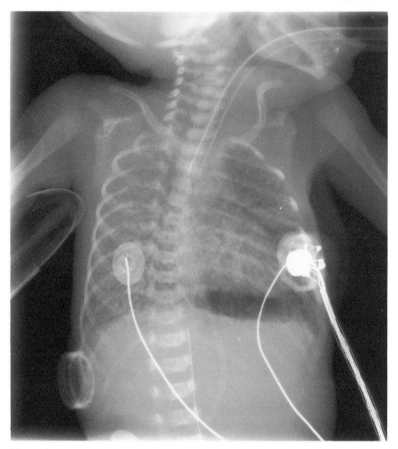

Figure 27

Technical comments

Exposure satisfactory (spine visible through heart shadow); inspiratory film and overinflated (10 posterior rib ends visible above the right diaphragm); marked rotation to the left (anterior rib ends asymmetrically placed and posterior ribs appear longer on the left); not lordotic (upper ribs appear to curve forwards and downwards); head facing the left.

Clinical equipment

Two ECG electrodes, a transcutaneous gas monitor probe/sensor and a spare base, endotracheal tube (ETT), nasogastric tube (NGT), umbilical arterial catheter (UAC) and right arm central venous line in situ.

Radiological interpretation

Apparent displacement of mediastinum and heart to the left is due to marked rotation. ETT tip at T3. Reticular pattern and mild pulmonary interstitial emphysema of both lung fields. Increased translucency of left lower lung field and flattened left diaphragm suggestive of a probable left anterior pneumothorax but there could also be gas in the pericardial cavity. NGT tip not shown. No gas in abdomen. UAC tip at T11. Central venous line in subclavian vein.

Conclusion

Probable left anterior pneumothorax and possible pneumopericardium with bilateral pulmonary interstitial emphysema in a preterm infant on intensive care.

Suggest left lateral view of chest, infant lying supine, using a horizontal beam to confirm anterior pneumothorax.

CASE STUDY 24: AP VIEW OF PRETERM CHEST AND UPPER ABDOMEN

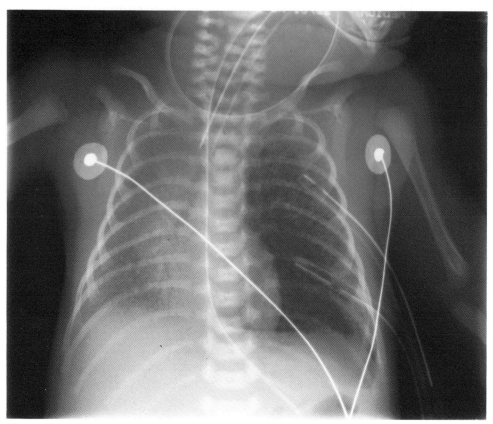

Figure 28

Technical comments

Exposure satisfactory (spine visible through heart shadow); overinflated (10
posterior rib ends visible above right diaphragm); not rotated (anterior rib ends
symmetrically placed); not lordotic (upper ribs appear to curve forwards and
downwards); head facing to the left. The loop of nasogastric tube and the ECG lead
should have been moved from the field of interest.

Clinical equipment

Two ECG electrodes, endotracheal tube (ETT), nasogastric tube (NGT) and two left
chest drains in situ.

Radiological interpretation

Mediastinum and heart displaced to the right. ETT tip at T3–4. Left mid-lung field
pulmonary interstitial emphysema; increased translucency of left lung field
indicates a partially drained left pneumothorax. Air bronchogram is clearly visible
in the compressed/collapsed/consolidated right lung field. NGT in stomach.

Conclusion

Left pulmonary interstitial emphysema and left anterior tension pneumothorax
probably due to respiratory distress syndrome in a preterm infant on intensive
care. The tips of the left chest drains are probably placed posteriorly and not
draining the anterior tension pneumothorax.
  Suggest:

1. Left lateral view of chest in dorsal decubitus position (lying supine) with a
   horizontal x-ray beam (see Figures 4 and 29) to confirm anterior pneumothorax
   and review the position of the tips of the chest drains.

2. Readjustment of position of tips of left chest drains.

Differential diagnosis – nosocomial infection in particular group B streptococcus.
Infection screen required.

CASE STUDY 25: LATERAL VIEW OF CHEST AND ABDOMEN OF PRETERM INFANT IN DORSAL DECUBITUS (SUPINE) POSITION WITH HORIZONTAL BEAM PROJECTION

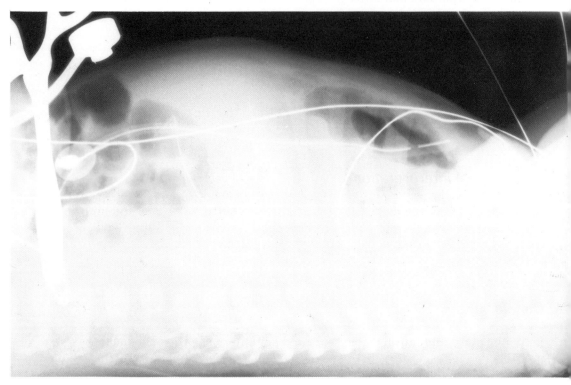

Figure 29

Technical comments

Exposure satisfactory (see page 5); not significantly rotated. X-ray field too large, abdomen irradiated unneccessarily. Multiple ECG leads should have been removed from field of interest.

Clinical equipment

Two ECG electrodes, multiple ECG leads, a transcutaneous gas monitor probe/sensor, a chest drain with attached Spencer Wells forceps, and nasogastric tube (NGT) in situ.

Radiological interpretation

Retrosternal collection of air due to an anterior pneumothorax. Chest drain well placed. NGT tip in stomach. Bowel gas shadows appear normal. No evidence of free gas in abdomen (see pages 154–5).

Conclusion

Anterior pneumothorax in a preterm infant on intensive care. Chest drain well placed.

CASE STUDY 26 (A SERIES OF FOUR FILMS): AP VIEW OF PRETERM CHEST AND UPPER ABDOMEN

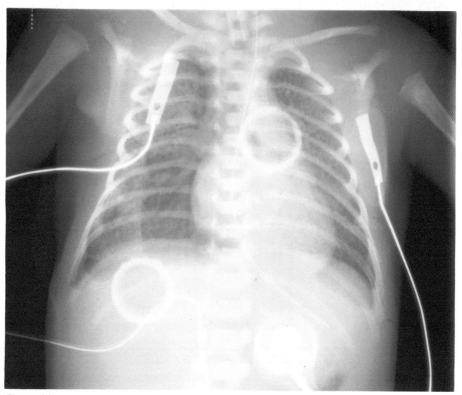

Figure 30a

LATERAL VIEW OF CHEST OF PRETERM INFANT IN DORSAL DECUBITUS POSITION (LYING ON BACK) WITH HORIZONTAL BEAM PROJECTION

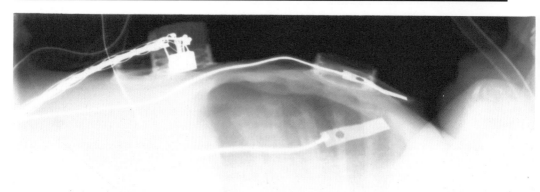

Figure 30b

Technical comments

Figure 30a – Exposure satisfactory (spine visible through heart shadow); inspiratory film with overexpanded chest (10 posterior rib ends visible above right diaphragm); slight rotation (anterior rib ends asymmetrically placed); not lordotic (upper ribs appear to curve forwards and downwards).

Figure 30b – Satisfactory exposure.

Clinical equipment

Two ECG electrodes, a transcutaneous gas monitor probe/sensor and several bases, an endotracheal tube (ETT) and a nasogastric tube (NGT) in situ. Right chest ECG electrode should have been resited to the right shoulder.

Radiological interpretation

Figure 30a – Mediastinum and heart not displaced. ETT tip at T1. Possible right anterior pneumothorax adjacent to right border of heart (not identified on this or lateral view (Figure 30b) at the time). Reticular shadowing to both lung fields which are overexpanded, probably due to high ventilator pressures.

Figure 30b – No obvious retrosternal collection of gas.

Figure 30c,d – Pneumothorax clearly demonstrated overleaf.

Conclusion

Small right pneumothorax and probable hyaline membrane disease in a preterm infant on intensive care.

Note

■ Small pneumothoraces may be demonstrated best on an AP view with the infant in the lateral decubitus position (affected side up) and a horizontal x-ray beam projection.

CASE STUDY 26 (CONTINUED)**: AP VIEWS OF CHEST OF PRETERM INFANT IN LATERAL DECUBITUS POSITION** (LYING ON LEFT SIDE/RIGHT SIDE UP) **WITH HORIZONTAL BEAM PROJECTION**

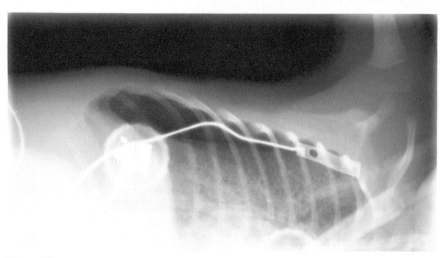

Figure 30c

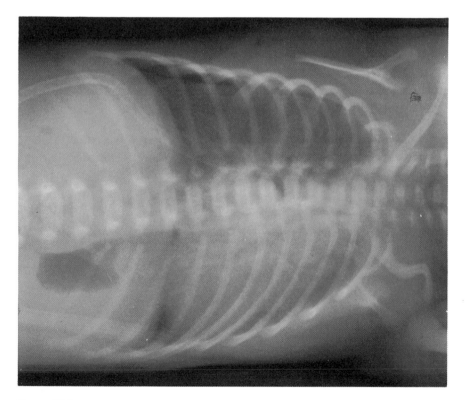

Figure 30d

Technical comments

Exposure satisfactory (spine visible through heart shadow); Figure 30c overexpanded chest (almost 10 posterior rib ends visible above right diaphragm), Figure 30d inspiratory film (9 posterior rib ends visible above right diaphragm); Figure 30d rotated to the left (anterior rib ends asymmetrically placed and posterior ribs appear longer on the left); Figure 30c lordotic (upper ribs horizontal), Figure 30d not lordotic (upper ribs appear to curve forwards and downwards). Figure 30c ECG lead should have been cleared from field of interest.

Clinical equipment

Figure 30c – ECG electrode and lead, transcutaneous blood gas monitor probe/sensor and separate base, nasogastric tube (NGT) and endotracheal tube (ETT) in situ.

Figure 30d – Right chest drain in situ.

Radiological interpretation

Figure 30d – mediastinum and heart rotated to the left. Both films show a small pneumothorax which was not visible on the projections shown in Figure 30a and b.

Conclusion

Small pneumothorax in a preterm infant.

Note

- Small pneumothoraces may be revealed best on an AP view with the infant in the lateral decubitus position (affected side uppermost) and a horizontal x-ray beam projection.

CASE STUDY 27 (A SERIES OF FOUR FILMS): AP VIEWS OF PRETERM CHEST AND UPPER ABDOMEN

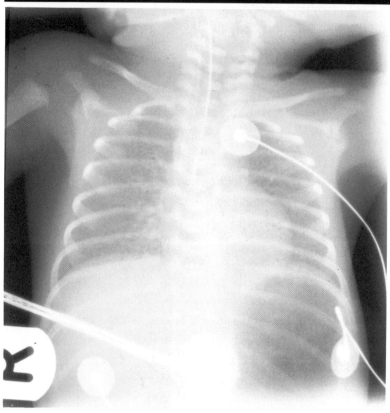

Figure 31a

Technical comments

Figure 31a underexposed relative to Figure 31b making comparison difficult (note difference in visibility of spine through heart shadow); Figure 31a expiratory film (7 posterior rib ends visible above the right diaphragm) and Figure 31b inspiratory film (9 posterior rib ends visible above the right diaphragm); Figure 31a not rotated, Figure 31b rotated to the right (anterior rib ends asymmetrically placed, and posterior ribs appear longer on the right); not lordotic (upper ribs appear to curve downwards and forwards); head facing right.

Clinical equipment

Figure 31a – Three ECG electrodes, a transcutaneous gas monitor probe/sensor, and an endotracheal tube (ETT) in situ.

Figure 31b – Two ECG electrodes, a transcutaneous gas monitor base, a nasogastric tube (NGT) and an endotracheal tube (ETT) in situ.

Radiological interpretation

Mediastinum and heart not displaced. ETT tip at T5 and probably in right main

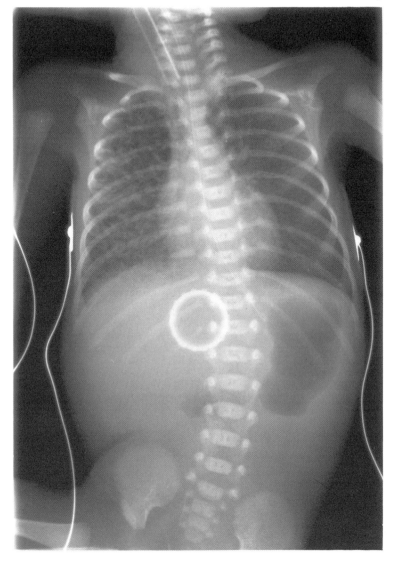

Figure 31b

bronchus (Figure 31a), withdrawn to T1 (Figure 31b). Appearance of lung fields in Figure 31a is due to underexposure and expiratory film whereas in Figure 31b it is normal in the left lung/chest and shows widespread pulmonary interstitial emphysema in the right lung/chest. The gross distension of the stomach with air (Figure 31a) has been relieved by an NGT (Figure 31b).

Conclusion

Iatrogenic pulmonary interstitial emphysema of right lung in a preterm infant on intensive care.

Note

 See pages 10 (gas leaks) and 239 (catheters/tubes).

CASE STUDY 27 (CONTINUED): AP VIEWS OF PRETERM CHEST AND UPPER ABDOMEN

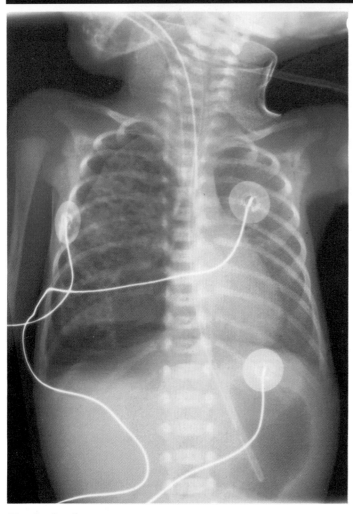

Figure 31c

Technical comments

Exposure satisfactory (spine visible through heart shadow); inspiratory film with overexpanded chest (10/11 posterior rib ends visible above the right diaphragm); Figure 31c not significantly rotated (anterior rib ends symmetrically placed); Figure 31d rotated to the right (anterior rib ends not symmetrically placed and posterior ribs appear longer on the right); not lordotic (upper ribs appear to curve downwards and forwards); head facing to the right. ECG leads should have been cleared from field of interest.

Clinical equipment

Three ECG electrodes, endotracheal tube (ETT), a nastogastric tube (NGT) and neck strapping in situ.

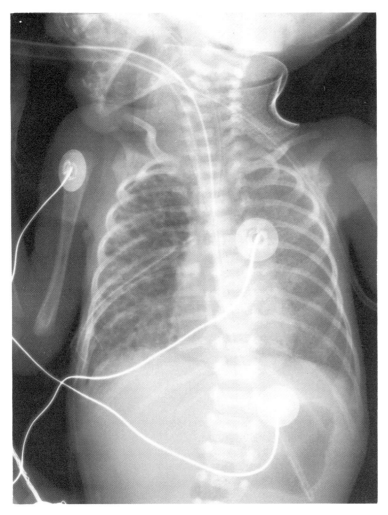

Figure 31d

Radiological interpretation

Mediastinum and heart: Figure 31c displaced to the left, Figure 31d not displaced. ETT tip at T4, i.e. at bifurcation of trachea. Widespread right lung pulmonary interstitial emphysema with right early tension pneumothorax (Figure 31c) – overexpanded, overinflated right chest with displaced mediastinum/heart, flattened diaphragm and splaying ribs. Tension pneumothorax relieved by chest drain (Figure 31d) but chest remains overexpanded/inflated suggestive of excessive ventilator pressures. NGT passes into stomach. Liver and bowel gas shadows appear normal.

Conclusion

Right-sided tension pneumothorax and widespread right lung pulmonary interstitial emphysema in a preterm infant on intensive care. The normal left lung and the probable high ventilator pressures suggest an originally iatrogenic cause.

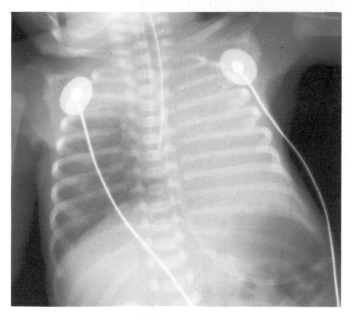

Figure 32a

Technical comments

Figure 32a underexposed relative to Figure 32b (clarity of soft tissues of neck and shoulders); expansion/inflation grossly pathological in both Figures 32a and b (see radiological interpretation); Figure 32a rotated to the left and Figure 32b rotated to the right (note position of anterior rib ends and compare length of posterior ribs on each side); not lordotic (upper ribs appear to curve forwards and downwards); Figure 32a head slightly facing right and Figure 32b head facing forwards. ECG leads should have been cleared from field of interest.

Clinical equipment

Figure 32a – Two ECG electrodes, endotracheal tube (ETT) and nasogastric tube (NGT) in situ.

Figure 32b – Two ECG electrodes, endotracheal tube (ETT), nasogastric tube (NGT), chest drain and right arm central venous line (CVL) in situ.

ECG electrodes should always be placed on shoulders where they will not obscure lung fields.

Radiological interpretation

Mediastinum and heart rotated and grossly displaced to the left in Figure 32a and indistinctly outlined in Figure 32b. Figure 32a: the ETT tip is at T7 in right lower

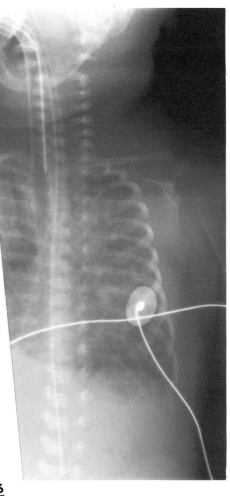

Figure 32b

upper lobe collapse and left lung collapse. Figure 32b: ·awn to T2. Both lungs now grossly overinflated (12)ve diaphragms). Bilateral patchy consolidation and ysema with a drained right pneumothorax. NGT ip in right subclavian vein.

llapse and left lung collapse followed by bilateral sema and a drained right pneumothorax in a ire (see Figure 32c and d).

1 239 (catheters/tubes).

CASE STUDY 28 (CONTINUED): AP VIEWS OF PRETERM CHEST

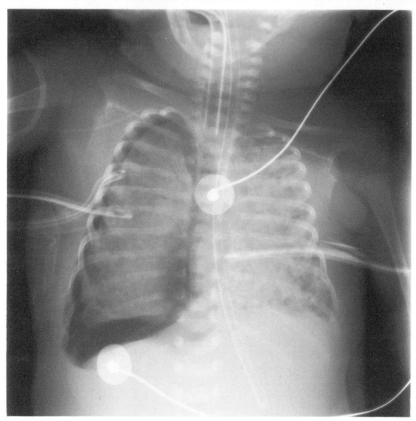

Figure 32c

Technical comments

Exposure satisfactory and comparable (spine visible through heart shadow); expansion/inflation grossly pathological in Figures 32c and d (see radiological interpretation); Figure 32c slightly rotated, Figure 32d not rotated (note position of anterior rib ends and compare length of posterior ribs on each side); not lordotic (upper ribs appear to curve forwards and downwards); head facing forward.

Clinical equipment

Figure 32c – Two ECG electrodes, endotracheal tube (ETT), nasogastric tube (NGT), three chest drains and right arm central venous line (CVL) in situ. The ECG electrodes should be removed from field of interest.

Figure 32d – Two ECG electrodes, endotracheal tube (ETT), nasogastric tube (NGT), six chest drains and right arm central venous line (CVL) in situ.

Radiological interpretation

Mediastinum and heart grossly displaced to the left in Figure 32c, with the ETT tip at T2. Right tension pneumothorax – gross right chest overinflation (12 posterior rib ends visible above right diaphragm) with mediastinum/heart

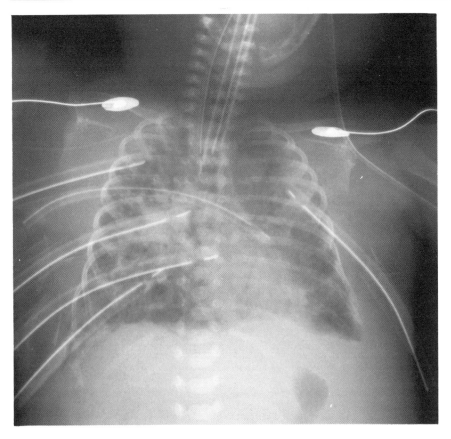

Figure 32d

displaced to the left, flattened diaphragm and splaying of ribs. Gas will collect anterior to the collapsed/consolidated right lung. The two chest drains should be manipulated to resite tips anteriorly (apex and base) in the collection of gas. Patchy collapse consolidation of left lung. Figure 32d: the ETT at T3. Overexpansion (?inflation) of right and left chest (flattened diaphragms and 10/11 posterior rib ends visible above diaphragms). Multiple right bullous lesions and bilateral patchy consolidation suggestive of bronchopulmonary dysplasia. Four right chest drains and two left chest drains in situ (St Sebastian). Infant now grossly oedematous. NGT tip in stomach (Figure 32c) and in oesophagus (Figure 32d). CVL tip in right subclavian vein.

Conclusion

Figure 32c – Inadequately drained right tension pneumothorax and patchy collapse consolidation of left lung in preterm infant on intensive care.

Figure 32d – Bilateral drained pneumothoraces and severe bronchopulmonary dysplasia in a grossly oedematous (renal failure) infant on intensive care.

Note

■ **This was a case of iatrogenic disease originally caused by the misplacement of the ETT tip in the right lower lobe bronchus** (see page 239).

CASE STUDY 29: AP VIEW OF PRETERM CHEST AND ABDOMEN

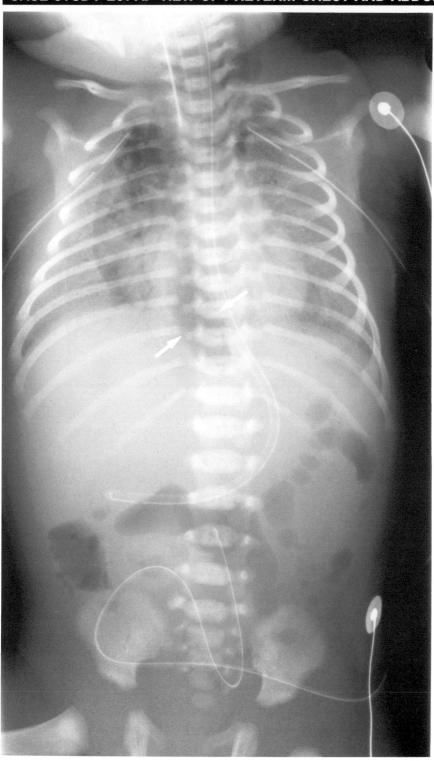

Figure 33

Technical comments

Exposure satisfactory (spine visible through heart shadow); inspiratory film (9 posterior rib ends visible above the right diaphragm); marked rotation to the right (anterior rib ends asymmetrically placed and posterior ribs appear longer on the right); lordotic (right upper ribs appear horizontal).

Clinical equipment

Two ECG electrodes, endotracheal tube (ETT), nasogastric tube (NGT), two chest drains and umbilical arterial catheter (UAC) in situ.

Radiological interpretation

Mediastinum and heart not displaced. ETT tip at T2. Retrosternal collection of gas alongside right mediastinum and anterior to the heart (arrows) with probable right anterior pneumothorax. The right chest drain is poorly placed to drain this pneumothorax. Left small apical pneumothorax with well-placed chest drain. Gas in left side of neck – leak from mediastinum or introduced by left chest drain. NGT tip in first part of duodenum. UAC tip at L4. Liver and bowel gas shadows appear normal. No gas in rectum.

Conclusion

Bilateral pneumothoraces, pneumomediastinum, surgical emphysema and severe probable hyaline membrane disease in a preterm infant on intensive care. The right anterior pneumothorax is inadequately drained.

Suggest right lateral view of chest with infant in dorsal decubitus position (supine) and horizontal x-ray beam projection to confirm anterior pneumothorax and localize tip of drain (see Figure 29).

CASE STUDY 30: AP VIEW OF PRETERM CHEST AND UPPER ABDOMEN

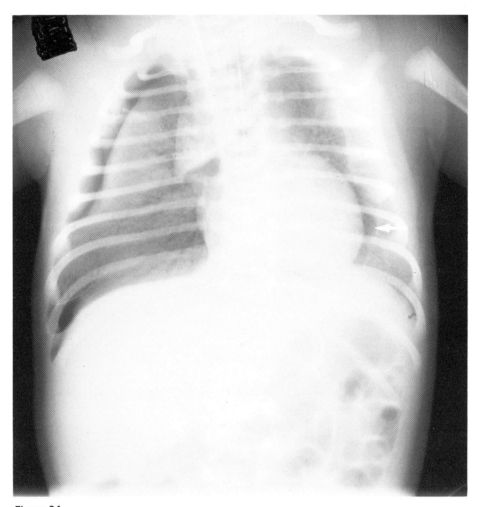

Figure 34

Technical comments

Underexposed (difficult to visualize spine through the heart shadow); inspiratory film (9 posterior rib ends visible above the right diaphragm); significantly rotated to the right (anterior rib ends asymmetrically placed and asymmetry of rib cage – right posterior ribs appear longer); markedly lordotic (upper ribs appear to curve forwards and upwards).

Clinical equipment

Endotracheal tube (ETT) and nasogastric tube (NGT) in situ.

Radiological interpretation

Mediastinum and heart not displaced. Possible pneumopericardium (arrow). ETT tip at T2. Right pneumothorax with no evidence of tension. Ground glass appearance to both lungs typical of hyaline membrane disease. Lungs have decreased compliance (stiff/consolidated/poorly aerated) and therefore have limited ability to collapse with the leakage of gas into the pleural cavity. The thymus is revealed by the pneumomediastinum giving the sail sign. NGT tip at pylorus. Liver and bowel shadows appear normal.

Conclusion

Right pneumothorax, possible pneumopericardium and severe probable hyaline membrane disease in a preterm infant on intensive care.

Note

■ The thymic notch, sail sign, may be present in the absence of a pneumothorax or pneumomediastinum.

■ The thymus shrinks rapidly under conditions of neonatal stress.

CASE STUDY 31: AP VIEW OF TERM CHEST AND UPPER ABDOMEN

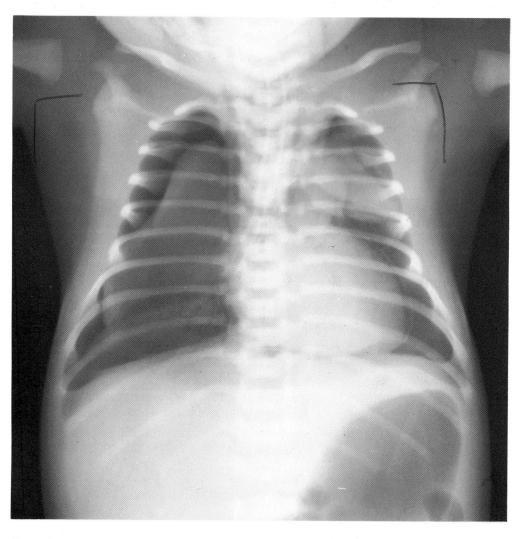

Figure 35

Technical comments

Exposure satisfactory (spine visible through heart shadow); inspiration/expansion grossly pathological (see radiological interpretation); not rotated (anterior rib ends symmetrically placed); not lordotic (upper ribs appear to curve forwards and downwards); head facing forwards.

Clinical equipment

Shouldered (Coles) endotracheal tube (ETT) in situ.

Radiological interpretation

Mediastinum and heart not displaced. ETT tip at T7 in right lower lobe bronchus. Bilateral pneumothoraces, pneumopericardium and pneumomediastinum. Thymus outlined on the left by gas.

Conclusion

Iatrogenic pneumopericardium and bilateral pneumothoraces in a term infant. Suggest:

1. Immediate withdrawal of ETT tip to T2/3.

2. Immediate insertion of butterfly needles into right and left chest.

3. Adequate ventilation and resuscitation.

4. Insertion of right and left chest drains.

5. Repeat chest x-ray.

Note

▨ A large collection of gas in the pericardial cavity may cause cardiac tamponade and may require emergency drainage.

CASE STUDY 32: AP VIEWS OF PRETERM CHEST

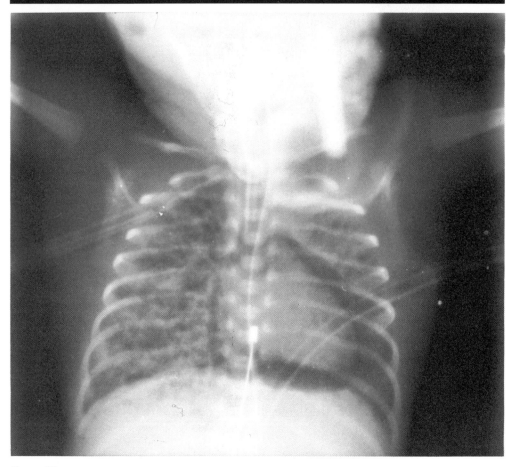

Figure 36a

Technical comments

Figure 36a – Exposure satisfactory (spine visible through heart shadow); inspiratory film (9 posterior rib ends visible above right diaphragm); not rotated (anterior rib ends symmetrically placed); slightly lordotic (upper ribs horizontal); head facing forwards; poor collimation of x-ray.

Figure 36b – Exposure satisfactory.

Clinical equipment

Figure 36a – Endotracheal tube (ETT), two chest drains, umbilical arterial catheter/electrode (UAC) and nasogastric tube (NGT) in situ.

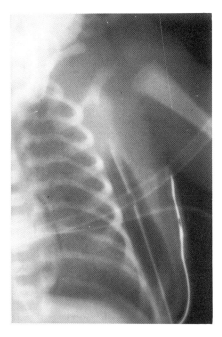

Figure 36b

Figure 36b. ECG electrode and chest drain in situ.

Radiological interpretation

Figure 36a – ETT tip at T4 at bifurcation of trachea. Massive pneumopericardium present. Irregular areas of opacification with adjacent areas of translucency affecting whole of both lung fields. Area of translucency over left costophrenic angle – possible pneumothorax. Tip of right chest drain at apex. Tip of left chest drain misplaced with tip at level of T10. UAC tip at T8. NGT passing down, presumably into stomach.

Figure 36b – Gas in subcutaneous tissues, surrounding misplaced/dislodged chest drain (vertical). Gas also in the brachial vein and in the pericardial cavity.

Conclusion

Severe bronchopulmonary dysplasia in a preterm infant on intensive care complicated by a left pneumothorax, surgical emphysema, air/gas embolus in the brachial vein and massive pneumopericardium probably causing cardiac tamponade.

CASE STUDY 33: AP VIEW OF PRETERM CHEST AND UPPER ABDOMEN

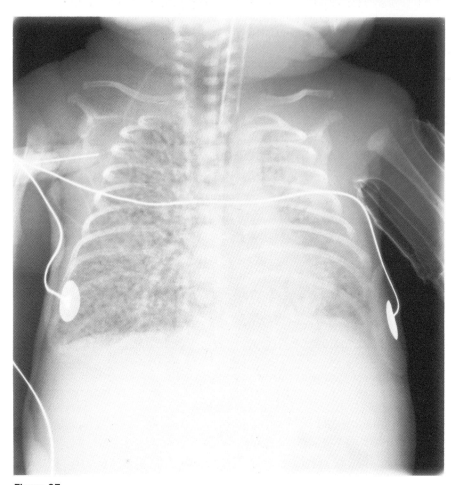

Figure 37

Technical comments

Exposure satisfactory (spine visible through heart shadow); inspiratory film and overexpanded (11 posterior rib ends visible above right diaphragm and flat diaphragms); some rotation to the left (posterior ribs appear longer on the left and endotracheal tube displaced to the left); not lordotic (upper ribs appear to curve forwards and downwards). Left ECG lead should have been moved from field of interest.

Clinical equipment

Two ECG electrodes, endotracheal tube (ETT), nasogastric tube (NGT), central venous line and blood pressure monitor cuff in situ.

Radiological interpretation

Mediastinum and heart displaced to the left. ETT tip at T2. Severe pulmonary interstitial emphysema and early changes of broncholpulmonary dysplasia in both lungs. Gross overexpansion of right lung causing displacement of the mediastinum and heart, compression of the left lung and flattening of the right diaphragm. The degree of displacement appears increased due to rotation. Right central venous line in superior vena cava. Tip cannot be seen but could be located by contrast medium (see page 267). Pocket of air seen in upper oesophagus.

Conclusion

Early bronchopulmonary dysplasia complicating severe pulmonary interstitial emphysema in a preterm infant on intensive care.

Note

See page 10 (air/gas leaks and bronchopulmonary dysplasia).

CASE STUDY 34: AP VIEW OF CHEST AND UPPER ABDOMEN

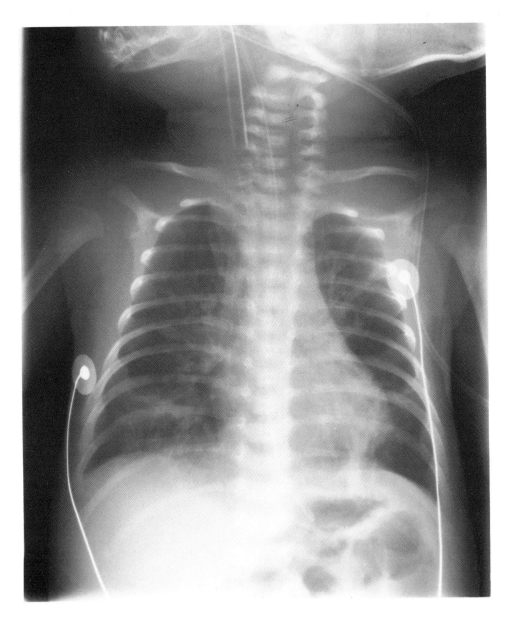

Figure 38 *This film was taken 4 weeks after birth.*

Technical comments

Exposure satisfactory (spine visible through heart shadow); overinflated (10 posterior rib ends visible on the right above the diaphragm); not rotated (anterior rib ends symmetrically placed); lordotic (upper ribs horizontal); head facing right for true positioning of endotracheal tube tip.

Clinical equipment

Two ECG electrodes, endotracheal tube (ETT) and nasogastric tube (NGT) in situ.

Radiological interpretation

ETT tip high. Overinflated chest giving the appearance of long thin heart, translucent lung fields and bilateral flat diaphragms. Regular bronchoalveolar architecture of both lung fields distorted by adjacent areas of alveolar collapse and emphysema with one or two large cysts and the appearance of air/gas trapping. Liver on the right. Stomach on the left. NGT tip in stomach.

Conclusion

Late bronchopulmonary dysplasia in a preterm infant (4 weeks after birth).

Note

■ See page 10 (gas leaks and bronchopulmonary dysplasia).

CASE STUDY 35: AP VIEW OF PRETERM CHEST AND UPPER ABDOMEN

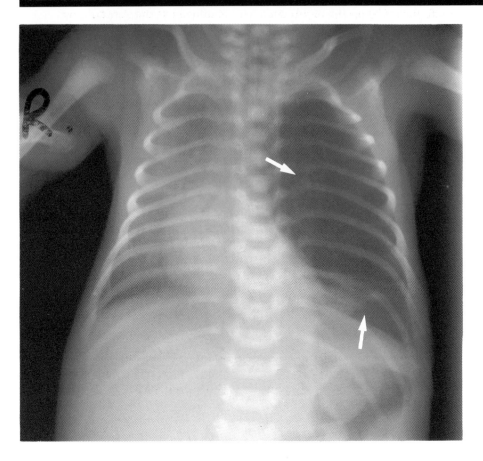

Figure 39

Technical comments

Exposure satisfactory (spine visible through heart shadow and lung detail visible); overinflated left chest (10 posterior rib ends visible above left diaphragm); not rotated (anterior rib ends symmetrically placed); not lordotic (upper ribs appear to curve forwards and downwards).

Clinical equipment

Catheter in oesophagus.

Radiological interpretation

Mediastinum and heart grossly displaced to the right. Increased translucency of left lung with faint lung markings (arrows) in left upper and lower-lung fields differentiates it from pneumothorax. Compression of left lower lung field and right lung. Left diaphragm flattened. Liver on the right. Stomach on the left. Catheter tip position not seen clearly.

Conclusion

Congenital lobar emphysema affecting left upper lobe.

If respiratory distress severe and worsening, consider selective intubation of right main bronchus and intermittent positive pressure ventilation.

CASE STUDY 36: AP VIEW AND RIGHT LATERAL VIEW OF CHEST AND UPPER ABDOMEN OF TERM INFANT IN ERECT POSITION WITH HORIZONTAL BEAM PROJECTION

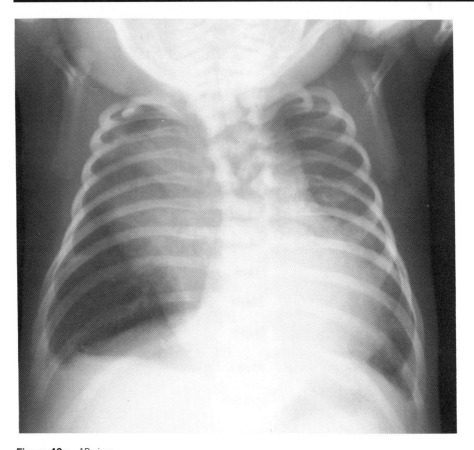

Figure 40a. *AP view.*

Technical comments

Figure 40a – Exposure satisfactory (spine just visible through heart shadow); overexpanded (10 posterior rib ends visible above right diaphragm); slight rotation to the right (anterior rib ends asymmetrically placed and posterior ribs appear longer on the right); not lordotic (upper ribs appear to curve forwards and downwards); head facing forwards.

Figure 40b – Exposure satisfactory, minimal rotation (anterior rib ends do not coincide).

Note: erect positioning unnecessary and hazardous.

Clinical equipment

Nil.

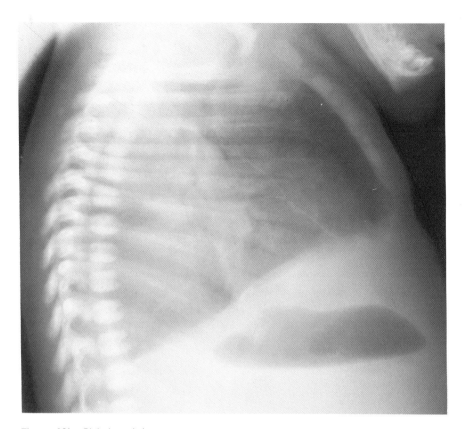

Figure 40b. *Right lateral view.*

Radiological interpretation

Figure 40a – Upper thoracic vertebral abnormalities present. Despite rotation to
the right, heart and mediastinum are displaced to the left by an opacity in the
right chest. Right lower lung field is translucent with lung markings. Part of
right diaphragm is flattened. Remaining visible left lung field and left
diaphragm appear normal.

Figure 40b – Posterior mediastinal mass with flattening of right posterior
diaphragm. Oblique fissure visible. Sternum not fused and lower thoracic
vertebrae are normal.

Upper abdomen in Figure 40a and b appears normal.

Conclusion

Vertebral abnormalities and a posterior mediastinal mass suggest a neurenteric cyst.

Note

▪ When examining the chest x-ray look for skeletal abnormalities (vertebral
abnormalities, 11 or 13 ribs) which are often clues to other associated
abnormalities.

CASE STUDY 37: AP VIEW OF CHEST AND UPPER ABDOMEN OF PRETERM INFANT IN SUPINE POSITION WITH VERTICAL BEAM PROJECTION

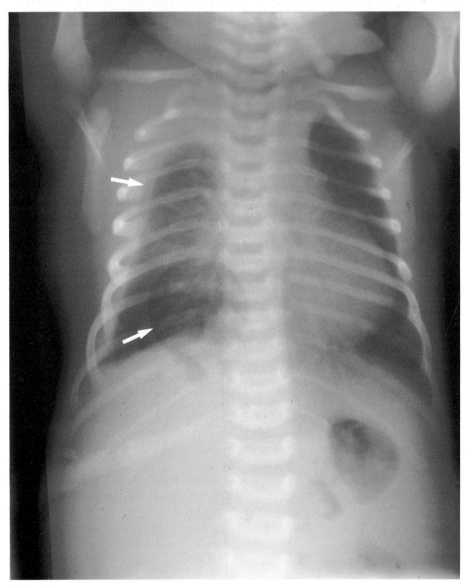

Figure 41

Technical comments

Exposure satisfactory (spine visible through heart shadow); inspiratory film (9 posterior rib ends visible above right diaphragm); rotated to the left (anterior rib ends asymmetrically placed and posterior ribs appear longer on the left); lordotic (upper ribs appear horizontal because arms raised).

Clinical equipment

Nil.

Radiological interpretation

Apparent displacement of heart and mediastinum to the left is partly due to rotation. Opacity in upper left medial lung field is mediastinum. Rest of left lung field appears normal. Opacity of right upper lung field extends caudally separating outer margin of right lung from inner aspect of right ribs and opacifying right costophrenic angle. Circular translucencies in upper (arrow) and lower (arrow) right lung fields. Liver on the right. Stomach on the left. Opacities over right abdomen probably artefacts.

Conclusion

Right-sided pleural effusion in a preterm infant. Upper right lung field circular translucency extends lateral to lung margin and needs further views to define. Lower right lung field circular translucency is due to incubator hole (see p. 5).

Suggest AP views of chest with infant in lateral decubitus position and horizontal beam projection: (1) right side down to confirm pleural effusion; (2) right side up to try to define the right upper lung field translucency.

CASE STUDY 38: AP VIEW OF CHEST OF PRETERM INFANT IN LATERAL DECUBITUS POSITION (LYING ON RIGHT SIDE WITH LEFT SIDE UP) WITH HORIZONTAL BEAM PROJECTION

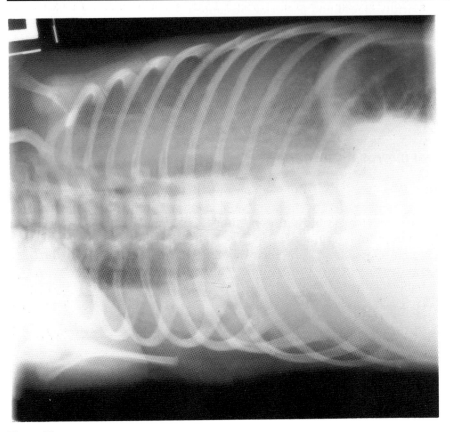

Figure 42

Technical comments

Note: this position of infant and projection of x-ray beam are recommended to demonstrate pleural effusion (see also Figure 30c and d – pneumothorax).

Exposure satisfactory (spine visible through heart shadow); markedly rotated to the left (anterior rib ends markedly asymmetrically placed and posterior ribs appear longer on the left); overexpanded chest (11 posterior rib ends visible on the left); not lordotic (upper rib ends appear to curve forwards and downwards).

Clinical equipment

Nil.

Radiological interpretation

Right chest large pleural effusion. Appearance of right lung crossing the midline and displacement of mediastinum and heart to the left is probably largely due to the marked rotation. Right diaphragm depressed/flattened.

Conclusion

Large right pleural effusion in a preterm infant.

CASE STUDY 39: AP VIEW OF CHEST AND ABDOMEN OF PRETERM INFANT

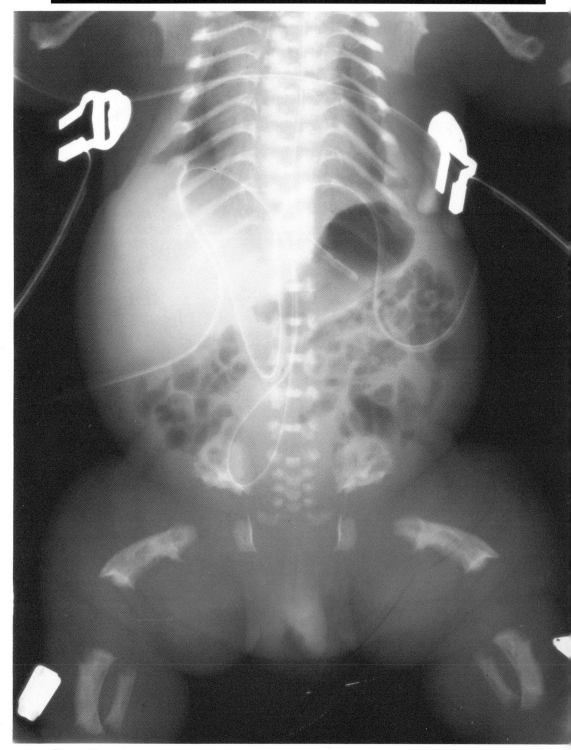

Figure 43

Technical comments

As this infant is obviously abnormal clinically, inclusion of legs and humeri on film is justified.

Clinical equipment

Nasogastric tube (NGT), umbilical arterial catheter (UAC) and umbilical venous catheter (UVC) in situ.

Radiological interpretation

Skeletal dysplasia. Abdomen – liver on the right and stomach on the left. NGT tip in stomach. UAC tip at T11. UVC tip over liver.

Conclusion

Asphyxiating thoracic dystrophy.

Note

Expert advice is required for the definitive diagnosis of the type of skeletal dysplasia and for genetic counselling which are beyond the purpose/scope of this manual.

NEONATAL HEART DISEASE

At birth the cardiovascular system makes the abrupt transition from the fetal circulatory pattern (systemic, pulmonary and placental circulations in parallel) to the neonatal pattern (systemic and pulmonary circulations in series). The expansion of the lungs and the rise in oxygen saturation of arterial blood are associated with a fall in the pulmonary vascular resistance (determined by medial arteriolar hypertrophy) and the pulmonary artery pressure; the latter may take 3–6 months to reach normal childhood levels. This fall is more rapid in the premature than the term infant and therefore **left to right shunts tend to reveal themselves earlier in the premature infant.**

Types

1. Non-structural

(a) Transient radiographic cardiomegaly is common and with severe cardiac failure may be associated with signs of pulmonary oedema.

(b) Causes: asphyxia; biochemical – hypoglycaemia, hypocalcaemia, electrolyte problems; infection; polycythaemia; high output cardiac failure – anaemia, arteriovenous malformations, etc; cardiac arrhythmias.

2. Persistent fetal circulation

(a) Frequency 1:1000 births.

(b) High pulmonary vascular resistance and pulmonary artery pressure with shunting from right to left across a persistent ductus arteriosus and foramen ovale, and on chest x-ray decreased pulmonary vascular markings.

3. Congenital heart disease

(a) Frequency 1:100 births with one in three being a serious structural abnormality.

(b) Alerting factors:

- family history of congenital heart disease;
- trisomy, e.g. Down's syndrome;
- dysmorphic infant.

(c) Presenting signs:

- murmurs
- cyanosis
- poor feeding
- cardiac failure

} may present early or after days/weeks

(d) Cyanotic congenital heart disease is suggested by:

- absence of above non-structural causes

- absence of signs of lung disease – $Paco_2 > 9.3$ kPa strongly suggests lung disease and a preductal $Pao_2 > 20$ kPa in 100% oxygen for 15 minutes excludes cyanotic congenital heart disease.

(e) Chest x-ray findings (see below).

Chest x-ray (AP view)

The chest x-ray is an essential initial investigation for respiratory distress and cyanosis and may help to differentiate heart from lung disease/pathology. **The radiological signs, though indicative, are often not diagnostic of the type of congenital heart disease, and other imaging techniques, e.g. echocardiography, are required for definitive diagnosis.**
A technically poor chest x-ray is useless for cardiovascular assessment:

- Incorrect exposure precludes assessment of the pulmonary vascular markings.

- Expiratory films cause crowding of pulmonary vascular markings and alter the cardiothoracic ratio and the heart shape.

- Rotated films alter heart shape (see Figures 47 and 54) and may alter lung translucency (see Figure 7).

- Lordotic films alter heart shape and falsely show heart apex elevated off the diaphragm.

A systematic approach is required to the interpretation of the chest x-ray:

1. *Assessment of the radiographic quality* (see introductory text to chest section) and *orientation*, i.e. right and left sides (see (5) below).

2. *Assessment of pulmonary vascular markings,* i.e. arterial supply; the normal pulmonary veins contribute little to the radiographic appearance.

(a) *Normal appearance* – pulmonary vasculature tapers and is visible to junction of middle and outer one-third of lung fields. In the middle third the adjacent arteries and bronchi are of similar diameter end on.

(b) *Decreased pulmonary vascular markings* (oligaemia) – implies right ventricular outflow tract obstruction, e.g. Fallot's tetralogy, pulmonary atresia. Pulmonary vasculature tapers and is visible to junction of inner and middle one-third of lung fields.

(c) *Increased pulmonary vascular markings* (plethora) – implies increased blood supply to the lungs caused by left to right shunt of at least 2:1 pulmonary to systemic flows. Pulmonary vasculature is prominent and visible to outer one-third of lung fields.

(d) *Pulmonary oedema* – implies impaired pulmonary venous drainage causing increased pulmonary venous pressure and extravasation of fluid into the interstitial tissues and alveoli. Caused by physical obstruction or failing left ventricular myocardium. Appearance is of distinct blood vessels replaced by diffuse haziness of lung fields.

3. *Assessment of great vessels and mediastinum* (Figure 44)

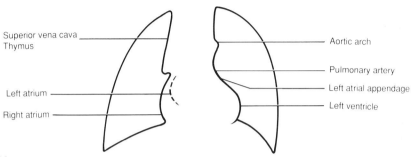

Figure 44

(a) Enlargement of superior vena cava and thymus causes widening of upper mediastinum but not displacement of trachea.

(b) Pulmonary artery may appear normal; prominent (convex) due to increased blood flow from left to right shunting at atrial or ventricular levels; 'absent' (concave) due to right ventricular outflow tract obstruction, e.g. Fallot's tetralogy, pulmonary atresia.

(c) The aortic arch is right sided in 30% of cases of Fallot's tetralogy, pulmonary atresia, truncus arteriosus and double outflow right ventricle.

4. *Assessment of the heart*

(a) Cardiomegaly is a cardiothoracic ratio of greater than 0.58 on adequate inspiration in a supine AP view with a focus–film distance of 1 metre. Unlike adults, the infant heart does not appear significantly larger on an AP than it does on a PA view.

(b) Position configurations other than a left-sided heart (laevocardia) and normal abdominal visceral locations (situs solitus) are abnormal. The heart also may be right sided (dextrocardia) or midline (mesocardia); these must be differentiated from displacement of the heart by lung/mediastinal disease, e.g. collapse, pneumothorax, lobar emphysema, mediastinal mass.

(c) Heart shape is not reliable for the diagnosis of the type of congenital heart disease.

5. *Assessment of the viscera*

(a) The abdominal visceral location may be situs solitus (normal, i.e. right-sided liver, left-sided stomach), situs inversus (right-sided stomach, left-sided liver) or situs ambiguus (unclear).

(b) It is normally indicative of the location of the right and left atrium – viscero-atrial concordance. Visceroatrial discordance (laevocardia and visceral inversion or dextrocardia and situs solitus) is associated with complex cyanotic congenital heart disease.

The upper abdomen should be included on chest films of infants with congenital heart disease so that the size of the liver can be noted, as it is a sensitive indicator of congestive cardiac failure. Enlargement may be confirmed on palpation of the abdomen.

Neonatal presentation of congenital heart disease

Abnormality	Presentation			Usual radiological appearance on chest x-ray
	Cyanosis	Murmur	Cardiac failure	
Cyanotic				
Transposition of great arteries *	Early		Frequent, early	30% of cases have classic appearance of narrow upper mediastinum, ovoid heart (egg on side). ↑ **Pulmonary vascular markings. 70% of cases have non-specific appearance**
Tetralogy of Fallot *	Early but may be delayed	Pulmonary stenotic murmer		Heart not enlarged. Develops boot shape later.↓ **Pulmonary vascular markings**. 30% have right aortic arch
Pulmonary atresia	Early			Heart size and shape variable. Concave pulmonary segment and ↓ **pulmonary vascular markings**
Tricuspid atresia *	Early	Pansystolic VSD in 50% of cases		Heart size and shape variable. Prominent right atrium and ↓ **pulmonary vascular markings**
Total anomalous venous return				
(a) Supracardiac/cardiac	Late	Pulmonary flow	Early	'Snowman heart' and ↑ **pulmonary vascular markings**
(b) Infradiaphragmatic	Early			Normal heart size, **pulmonary oedema**, ground glass appearance with no air bronchogram
Hypoplastic left heart syndrome *	Early	Pulmonary flow	Early	Cardiomegaly in 80% of cases. ↑ **pulmonary vascular markings**. Pulmonary venous congestion
Non-cyanotic – shunts				
Persistent ductus arteriosus (PDA)		Systolic to machinery	Late BUT MAY PRESENT EARLIER IN PRETERM INFANTS	Radiological features depend upon size of shunt. No changes until shunt is at least 2:1. Sequence of changes as follows: • ↑ **Pulmonary vascular markings** • Left atrial enlargement with ASD and VSD • Ventricular enlargement • Cardiac failure
Ventricular septal defect (VSD)	Late	Pansystolic		
Atrial septal defect (ASD)	Late	Pulmonary flow		
Atrioventricular canal defects	Late	Pulmonary flow		
Truncus arteriosis	Late	Systolic ± diastolic	Late	Biventricular hypertrophy, concave pulmonary artery segment. ↑ **Pulmonary vascular markings**. 40% have a right-sided aortic arch
Non-cyanotic – no shunts				
Coarctation of aorta		Interscapular systolic	Early or late	**Normal pulmonary vascular markings**. In cardiac failure – pulmonary oedema and non-specific cardiomegaly
Aortic stenosis		Systolic ejection	Early or late	
Pulmonary stenosis		Systolic ejection		**Normal pulmonary vascular markings**. Pulmonary artery segment may be convex because of post-stenotic dilatation

* May be dependent upon a persistent ductus arteriosus for adequate blood supply to lungs

The radiological features of some of these conditions are illustrated and described in the following case studies.

CASE STUDY 40: AP VIEW OF TERM CHEST AND ABDOMEN

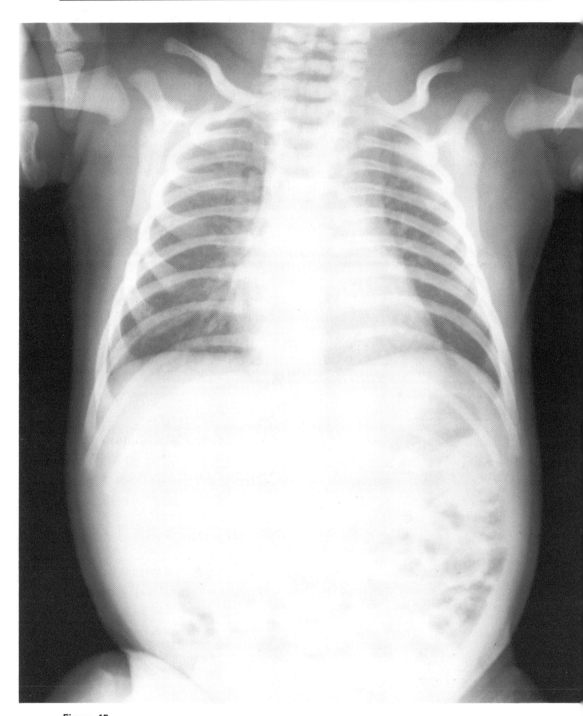

Figure 45

Technical comments

Slightly underexposed (spine just visible through heart shadow); inspiratory film (9 posterior rib ends visible above the right diaphragm); slightly rotated to the left (anterior rib ends asymmetrically placed and posterior ribs appear longer on the left); not lordotic (upper ribs appear to curve forwards and downwards). Assistant's fingers should not have been included in the field of exposure. Abdomen is included for assessment of liver size but this film is barely adequate for this purpose (underexposed).

Clinical equipment

Nil.

Radiological interpretation

Mediastinum and heart not displaced. Laevocardia. Heart shape normal and not enlarged (cardothoracic ratio 0.52). The pulmonary artery segment not clearly seen because of rotation and overlying thymus. Lung fields show normal to slightly increased vascular markings. Cervical ribs present. Liver on the right and stomach on the left (situs solitus). Liver not enlarged. Bowel gas shadows are poorly visualized but appear normal.

Conclusion

Probable increased blood flow to the lungs, with laevocardia, situs solitus and no radiological signs of cardiac failure in a term infant, suggests a left to right shunt which could be at atrial, ventricular or ductal levels.

CASE STUDY 41: AP VIEW OF TERM CHEST AND UPPER ABDOMEN

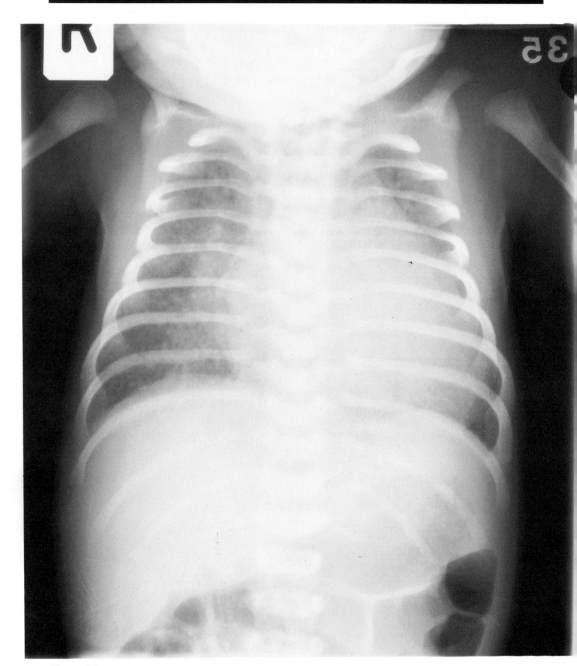

Figure 46

Technical comments

Slightly underexposed (spine just visible through heart shadow); partial inspiratory film but acceptable (8 posterior rib ends visible above the right diaphragm); not rotated (anterior rib ends symmetrically placed); slightly lordotic (upper ribs horizontal); head facing forwards.

Clinical equipment

Nil.

Radiological interpretation

Mediastinum and heart not displaced. Laevocardia. Cardiac enlargement (cardiothoracic ratio 0.68). Pulmonary artery segment convex. Lung fields show increased vascular markings (pulmonary plethora). Liver on the right and stomach on the left (situs solitus). Liver slightly enlarged. Bowel gas shadows appear normal.

Conclusion

Increased blood flow to the lungs (pulmonary plethora), enlarged heart and slight enlargement of liver (alerting one to the possibility of cardiac failure), laevocardia and situs solitus in a term infant suggests a large left to right shunt which could be at atrial, ventricular or ductal levels.

CASE STUDY 42: AP VIEW OF TERM CHEST AND UPPER ABDOMEN

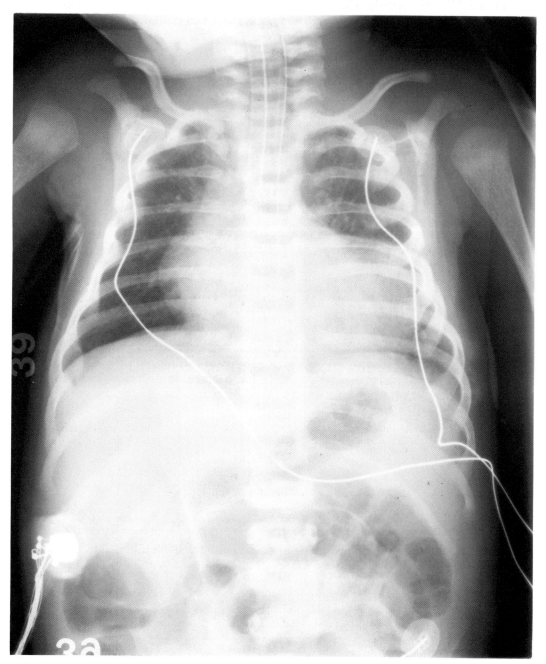

Figure 47

Technical comments

Exposure satisfactory (spine visible through heart shadow); partial inspiration but acceptable film (8 posterior rib ends visible above the right diaphragm); slightly rotated to the right (anterior rib ends asymmetrically placed); not lordotic (upper ribs appear to curve forwards and downwards); head facing to the right. ECG leads should have been cleared from the field of interest.

Clinical equipment

Three ECG electrodes, transcutaneous blood gas monitor probe/sensor, endotracheal tube (ETT) and nasogastric tube (NGT) in situ.

Radiological interpretation

ETT tip at T4, i.e. at bifurcation of trachea. Mediastinum and heart rotated/displaced to the right. Laevocardia. Cardiac enlargement (cardiothoracic ratio 0.68). Apex appears elevated and pulmonary segment concave – the pulmonary segment appearance is partly due to rotation. Normal vascular markings in the lung fields. Liver on the right and stomach on the left (situs solitus). Liver not enlarged. Some distended loops of bowel in the right abdomen. Otherwise bowel gas shadows appear normal. NGT tip at gastro-oesphageal junction.

Conclusion

Heart shape suggestive of Fallot's tetralogy in a term infant on intensive care. Slight deviation of trachea to the right suggests a left aortic arch.

Suggest ETT withdrawn by 1.5 cm and NGT inserted further.

Note

▨ 'Coeur en sabot' (boot-shaped heart) occurs in one-third of infants with tetralogy of Fallot.

CASE STUDY 43 (A SERIES OF TWO FILMS): AP VIEW OF PRETERM CHEST AND UPPER ABDOMEN

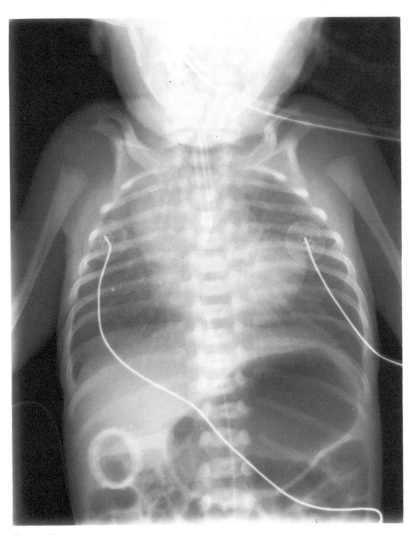

Figure 48a

Technical comments

Figure 48a – Exposure satisfactory (spine clearly visible through heart shadow); partial inspiratory film (8 posterior rib ends visible above the right diaphragm); not significantly rotated (anterior rib ends symmetrically placed); lordotic (upper ribs appear horizontal, see radiological interpretation); head facing forwards. ECG leads should have been removed from field of interest.

Clinical equipment

Figure 48a – Two ECG electrodes, transcutaneous blood gas monitor sensor base, endotracheal tube (ETT) and umbilical arterial catheter (UAC) in situ. ECG electrodes should have been placed outside field of interest, i.e. on shoulders.

Radiological interpretation

Figure 48a – Mediastinum and heart not displaced. Prominent right thymic shadow. Heart not enlarged (cardiothoracic ratio 0.55 even on this partial inspiratory film); the apex is elevated suggestive of right ventricular hypertrophy and the pulmonary artery segment is concave – 'coeur en sabot'. Thymic shadow partly fills in the concave pulmonary segment. ETT tip at T4 at bifurcation of trachea. Lung fields show normal to increased vascularity. 12 ribs present. UAC tip at T7. Liver on the right and stomach on the left. Gaseous distension of stomach.

Conclusion

See p. 115.

CASE STUDY 43 (CONTINUED): LATERAL VIEW OF PRETERM CHEST AND UPPER ABDOMEN

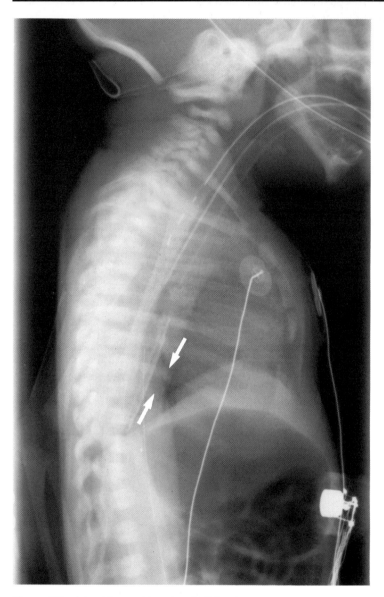

Figure 48b. *Infant lying on side and vertical X-ray beam.*

Technical comments

Figure 48b – Satisfactory exposure. ECG lead should have been removed from the field of interest, and baby's arms raised beside head, if possible.

Clinical equipment

Figure 48b – Two ECG electrodes, transcutaneous blood gas monitor sensor, endotracheal tube (ETT), umbilical arterial catheter (UAC) and nasogastric tube (NGT) in situ.

Radiological interpretation

Figure 48b – ETT tip at bifurcation of trachea. NGT tip in upper oesophagus. Heart and lungs appear normal. Sternum not fused (common in congenital heart disease). Gas in lower oesophageal pouch (arrows), stomach (distended) and bowel.

Conclusion

Preterm infant with a heart shape suggestive of tetralogy of Fallot but without pulmonary oligaemia, which suggests a significant left to right shunt, probably from the aorta to the pulmonary arteries; and oesophageal atresia with a fistula between the trachea and the lower oesophageal pouch.

Suggest:

1. Withdrawal of ETT by 1 cm.

2. Insertion of Replogle tube and continuous aspiration of blind upper oesophageal pouch.

3. Immediate transfer to a neonatal cardiac/surgical unit.

Note

■ Boot-shaped heart occurs in one-third of infants with tetralogy of Fallot.

■ With lordotic views the heart apex may appear falsely elevated, mimicking right ventricular hypertrophy.

■ Normal course of UAC on lateral view (see page 239).

CASE STUDY 44: AP VIEW OF TERM CHEST AND UPPER ABDOMEN

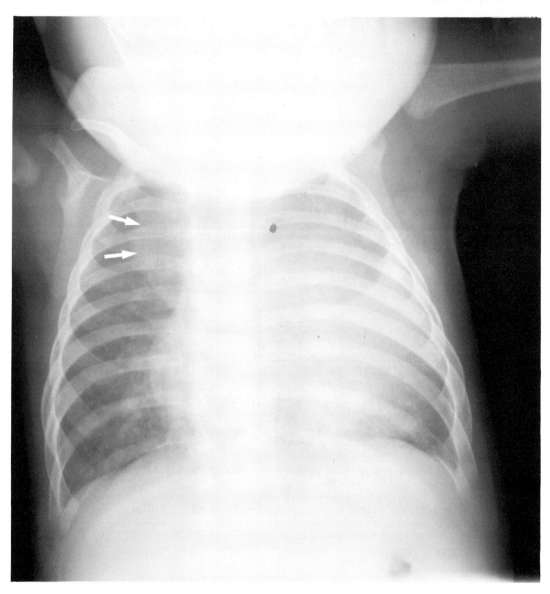

Figure 49

Technical comments

Slightly underexposed (spine hardly visible through the heart shadow); inspiratory film (10 posterior rib ends visible above the right diaphragm); rotated to the left (anterior rib ends asymmetrically placed and posterior ribs appear longer on the left); not lordotic (upper ribs appear to curve forwards and downwards); neck flexed and head facing forwards – padding under shoulders would allow neck extension and the face/head to be cleared from the upper lung fields.

Clinical equipment

Nil.

Radiological interpretation

Upper mediastinum widened (arrows). Laevocardia and cardiomegaly (cardiothoracic ratio unreliable because of rotation). Lung fields show increased vascularity (plethora). Liver on the right, stomach on the left (situs solitus). Black spot over left upper lung is an artefact.

Conclusion

'Snowman' appearance (widened upper mediastinum and cardiomegaly) and pulmonary plethora suggestive of type I total anomalous pulmonary venous drainage (TAPVD) in a term infant. Similar appearances can occur with a combination of a large thymus and a simple large left to right shunt (e.g. ventricular septal defect).

Type II TAPVD – pulmonary veins drain into coronary sinus/right atrium and therefore there is no widening of upper mediastinum.

Type III TAPVD – infradiaphragmatic pulmonary venous drainage is obstructed and results in pulmonary oedema and a small heart. An air bronchogram is not usually visible.

CASE STUDY 45: AP VIEW OF PRETERM CHEST AND UPPER ABDOMEN

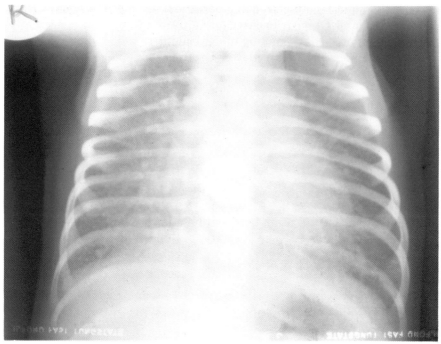

Figure 50

Technical comments

Exposure satisfactory (spine visible through heart shadow); inspiratory film (9 posterior rib ends visible above the right diaphragm); not significantly rotated (anterior rib ends symmetrically placed); slightly lordotic (upper ribs horizontal). Poor collimation – field size too restricted.

Clinical equipment

Nil.

Radiological interpretation

Mediastinum and heart not displaced. Laevocardia. Heart not enlarged (cardiothoracic ratio 0.57). Lung fields show markedly increased vascular markings (pulmonary plethora). Liver on the right, stomach on the left (situs solitus).

Conclusion

Marked pulmonary plethora with normal sized heart and situs solitus in a preterm infant suggestive of a large left to right shunt.

Differential diagnosis

- shunt at atrial/ventricular/ductal levels – non-cyanotic;
- total anomalous pulmonary venous drainage type II (narrow upper mediastinum) – cyanotic.

OESOPHAGEAL ATRESIA AND TRACHEO-OESOPHAGEAL FISTULA

Frequency

1:3500 births

Types

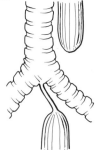

Oesophageal atresia
with lower pouch fistula (80-90%)

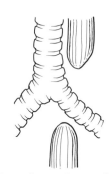

Oesophageal atresia
with no fistula (5-10%)

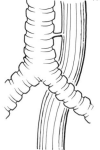

H fistula with
no atresia (5–8%)

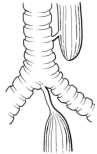

Oesophageal atresia with both
upper and lower pouch fistulae (1–3%)

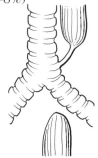

Oesophageal atresia
with upper pouch fistula only (1%)

Presentation

Oesophageal atresia ± fistula presents with:

- History of polyhydraminios.

- Excessive saliva and choking with inhalation of secretions.

- Cyanotic attacks on feeding – diagnosis should have been made before feeding.

- Inability to pass a stiff tube (French gauge 12) into stomach; passage of tube obstructed usually 10 cm from gum margin.

Note

- Fine tube may not get past cricopharyngeal sphincter to enter the oesophagus.

- Fistulous connection between tracheobronchial tree and lower oesophageal pouch suggested by gas in stomach.

- Absence of gas in stomach does not exclude a fistula especially in films taken early.

- 50% of cases have associated congenital malformations, e.g. duodenal atresia, VATER association (vertebral/vascular, anorectal, tracheo-oesophageal fistula, oesophageal atresia, radial/renal abnormalities).

- **Upper pouch can be continuously aspirated adequately ONLY with a REPLOGLE tube, without which aspiration into the lungs will occur** (see Figure 56).

- Radiographic centring on chest for AP and lateral views is essential for surgical assessment of extent of upper and lower oesophageal pouches.

- **The use of contrast media to define the upper pouch is dangerous and unnecessary.**

   Presentation of H fistula without atresia is characterized by recurrent episodes of aspiration and abdominal distension. Diagnosis may be made by the gradual withdrawal of an inserted nasogastric tube with the open end immersed in water: as the fistula is approached, air passing through the fistula into the oesophagus will bubble out of the immersed end of the catheter.

Technical note

It is essential to clear facial soft tissues and jaw from masking catheter curled in upper blind pouch (see Figure 57). Head should be turned to one side or cotton wool roll inserted under shoulders and neck extended.

CASE STUDY 46: AP VIEW OF CHEST OF TERM INFANT

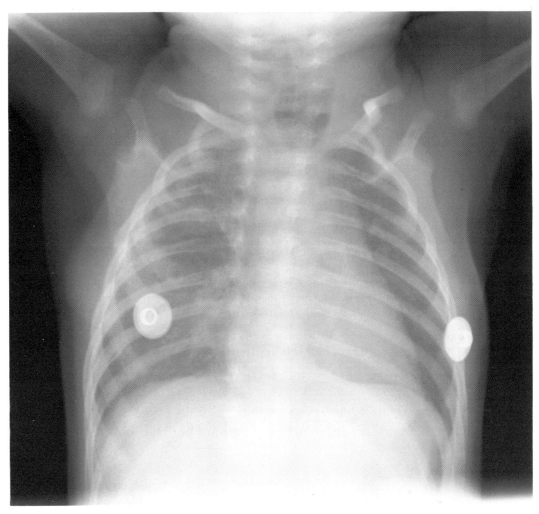

Figure 51

Technical comments

Exposure unsatisfactory (grey film, no lung detail); inspiratory film (9/10 posterior rib ends visible above the right diaphragm); rotated to the left (anterior rib ends asymmetrically placed and posterior ribs appear longer on the left); not lordotic (upper ribs appear to curve forwards and downwards); head facing forwards. Poor collimation of x-ray field: upper abdomen must be included to demonstrate presence/absence of gas in stomach.

Clinical equipment

Two ECG electrodes which should have been placed on shoulders away from the field of interest.

Radiological interpretation

Midline translucency overlying lower cervical/upper thoracic vertebrae and suggestive of the upper pouch of oesophageal atresia. Mediastinum and heart rotated to the left. Lung fields clear. No gas in abdomen.

Conclusions

Appearances of oesophageal atresia without fistula.

Suggest immediate insertion of Replogle tube, continuous suction clearance of secretions from upper oesophageal pouch and re-x-ray including upper abdomen.

CASE STUDY 47: AP AND LATERAL VIEWS OF PRETERM CHEST AND UPPER ABDOMEN

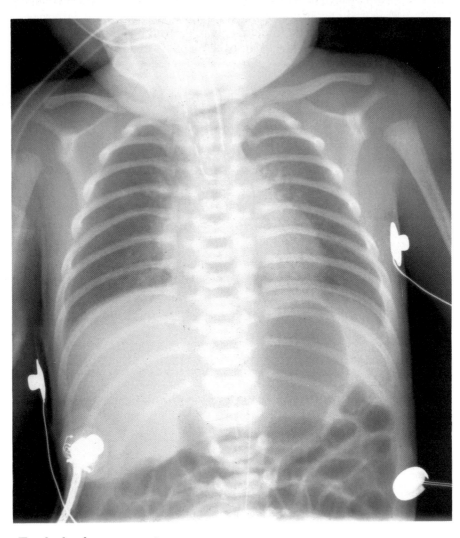

Figure 52a
AP view

Technical comments

Figure 52a – Exposure satisfactory (spine visible through heart shadow); expiratory film (7 posterior rib ends visible above the right diaphragm); not rotated (anterior rib ends symmetrically placed); slightly lordotic (upper ribs horizontal); head facing forwards.

Figure 52b – Underexposure and **malposition of arms obscure upper oesophagus**: the tube is not seen. To demonstrate its location is the reason for taking this film, so the infant has been irradiated to no purpose.

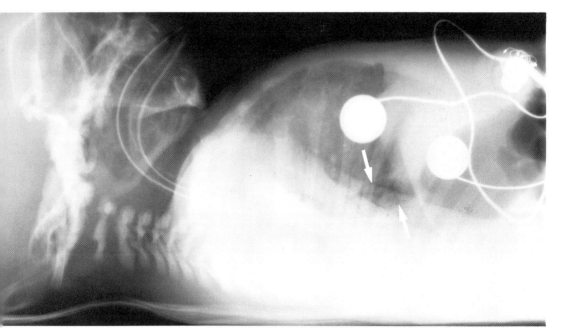

Figure 52b *Lateral view, in dorsal decubitus position with horizontal beam.*

Clinical equipment

Figures 52a and b – two ECG electrodes, a transcutaneous blood gas monitor probe/sensor, an endotracheal tube (ETT) and a double lumen Replogle tube in situ. Figure 52a – umbilical arterial catheter (UAC) in situ.

Radiological interpretation

Figure 52a – Mediastinum and heart normal. ETT tip at T3. Lung fields normal. Replogle tube tip at T4. Liver, spleen, stomach and bowel gas shadows normal. UAC tip curled at T12–L1.

Figure 52b – Gas in stomach and lower oesophageal pouch (arrows) clearly seen. Tip of UAC just on film. Tube in pouch **not** seen.

Conclusion

Oesophageal atresia with fistulous connection between the tracheobronchial tree and the lower oesophageal pouch in a preterm infant. UAC tip at level of renal arteries and could be in mouth of right renal artery.

Suggest withdraw catheter tip to L3.

CASE STUDY 48: LATERAL VIEW OF CHEST AND ABDOMEN OF PRETERM INFANT IN LATERAL DECUBITUS POSITION (RIGHT SIDE DOWN) WITH VERTICAL BEAM PROJECTION

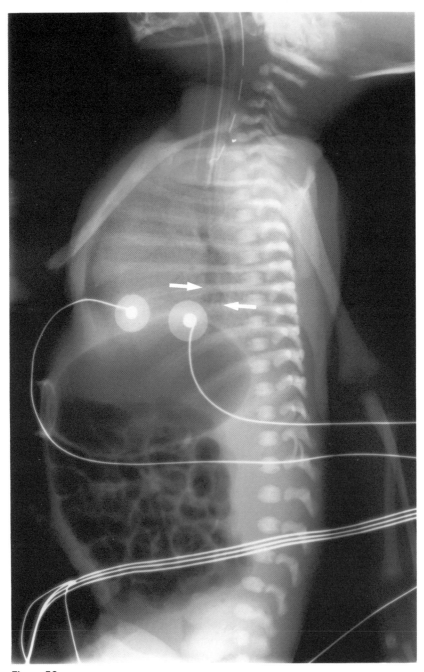

Figure 53

Technical comments

Exposure satisfactory for chest and abdomen (see page 5). Arms well cleared from area of interest (Replogle tube) – compare with Figure 48b and Figure 52b. Poor collimation of x-ray beam: field too large.

Clinical equipment

Two ECG electrodes, multiple leads, a transcutaneous blood gas monitor probe/sensor base, endotracheal tube (ETT) and Replogle tube in situ. ECG electrodes should have been placed away from the field of interest.

Radiological interpretation

ETT tip at T2. Replogle tube tip at T1. Translucencies of trachea and air in the lower oesophageal pouch clearly outlined (arrows). Gaseous distension of stomach and bowel indicates a fistulous connection between the tracheobronchial tree and lower oesophageal pouch. No evidence of free gas in peritoneum (see pages 154–5).

Conclusion

Oesophageal atresia and fistulous connection between the tracheobronchial tree and the lower oesophageal pouch in a preterm infant on intensive care.

CASE STUDY 49: AP VIEW OF PRETERM CHEST AND ABDOMEN

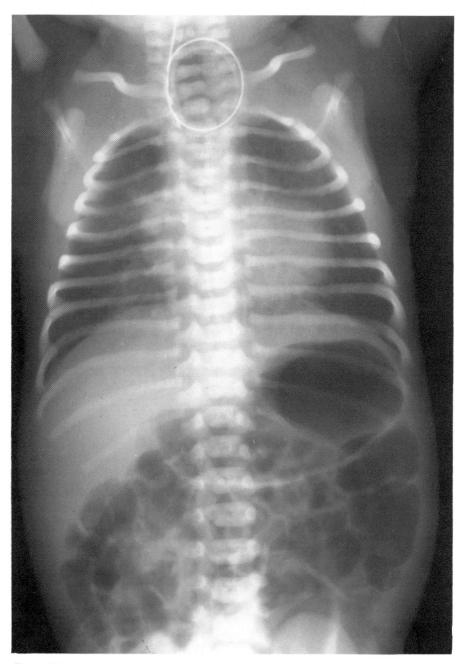

Figure 54

Technical comments

Exposure satisfactory (spine visible through heart shadow); inspiratory film (9 posterior rib ends visible above the right diaphragm); slightly rotated (asymmetry of rib cage); markedly lordotic (upper ribs appear to curve forwards and upwards) because arms held above head and centring is low. *Note:* correct collimation of lower abdomen to exclude gonads. Upper abdomen must always be included (as here) to show if gas present in stomach (i.e. fistula present).

Clinical equipment

Nasogastric tube (NGT) in situ.

Radiological interpretation

NGT is too fine and is curled up in dilated, gas filled upper oesophageal pouch. Liver on the right. Stomach on the left. Gas in distended stomach and bowel indicates a fistulous connection between the tracheobronchial tree and the lower pouch of the oesophagus. Lordotic position causes apparent elevation of heart apex off the diaphragm and rotation to the left gives concave pulmonary segment. This combination gives the erroneous appearance of a boot-shaped heart. Lung fields show normal vascularity. Horizontal fissure apparent. Increased opacification of right upper lung field probably due to aspiration.

Conclusion

Oesophageal atresia with a fistulous connection between the tracheobronchial tree and the lower oesophageal pouch and early signs of right upper lobe consolidation in a preterm infant.

Suggest immediate insertion of Replogle tube and continuous suction to prevent further aspiration.

CASE STUDY 50: LATERAL VIEW OF CHEST OF TERM INFANT IN LATERAL DECUBITUS POSITION WITH VERTICAL BEAM PROJECTION

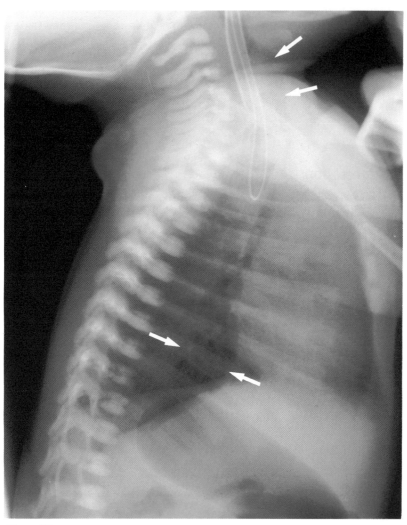

Figure 55

Technical comments

Exposure satisfactory: only slightly rotated (anterior rib ends do not coincide). Arms well cleared from field of interest.

Clinical equipment

Endotracheal tube (ETT) and oesophageal catheter in situ.

Radiological interpretation

ETT tip at C5 misplaced in oesphagus. Single lumen, fine bore catheter passing down oesophagus to T3 where it doubles back on itself – tip not on film. Gas in trachea (arrows) and gaseous distension of lower oesophageal pouch (arrows) and stomach.

Conclusion

Oesophageal atresia and fistulous connection between tracheobronchial tree and lower oesophageal pouch in an infant with an ETT in the oesophagus.

Note

■ Distance catheter passed may lead doctor to think, erroneously, it has passed into stomach.

■ Only stiff catheters should be used to avoid this error.

■ This infant's upper pouch is not being cleared of secretions and there is risk of aspiration.

Suggest correct repositioning of ETT and replacement of catheter with Replogle tube, continuous suction and AP chest x-ray to check correct positioning of tip of Replogle tube.

CASE STUDY 51: AP VIEW OF PRETERM CHEST AND UPPER ABDOMEN

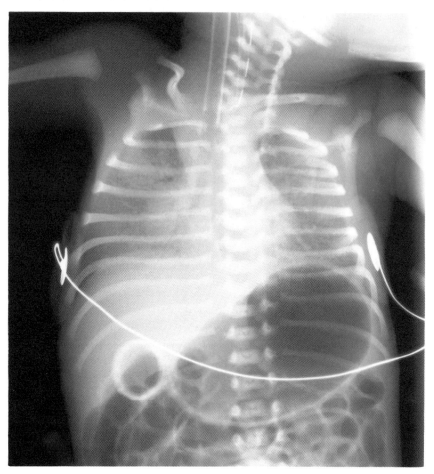

Figure 56

Technical comments

Exposure satisfactory (spine visible through heart shadow); expiratory film (7 posterior rib ends visible above the right diaphragm); grossly rotated to the right (posterior ribs appear markedly longer on the right); very lordotic (upper ribs appear to curve forwards and upwards); head turned to right.

Clinical equipment

Two ECG electrodes, transcutaneous blood gas sensor base, endotracheal tube (ETT) and double lumen Replogle tube in situ.

Radiological interpretation

Heart not enlarged. ETT tip at T1. Right upper lobe collapse and right mid-lung field consolidation due to aspiration. Replogle tube tip at C7. Gaseous distension of stomach and plentiful gas in bowel will exacerbate respiratory distress.

Conclusion

Oesophageal atresia and fistulous connection between the tracheobronchial tree and lower oesophageal pouch in a preterm infant on intensive care. Replogle tube inadequately inserted resulting in inadequate clearance of secretions from upper oesophageal pouch and aspiration causing right lung complications.

Suggest immediate further insertion of the Replogle tube with continuous effective clearance of secretions.

CASE STUDY 52: AP VIEW OF PRETERM CHEST AND ABDOMEN

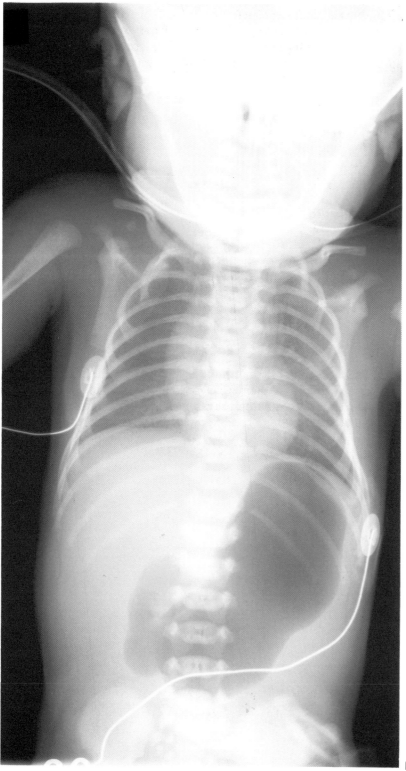

Figure 57

Technical comments

Exposure of preterm chest and abdomen satisfactory (see page 5); inspiratory film (9 posterior rib ends visible above the right diaphragm); not rotated (anterior rib ends symmetrically placed); not lordotic (upper ribs appear to curve forwards and downwards); head facing forwards and faciomaxillary structures overlying neck and lung apices. A small cotton-wool roll under shoulders would correct this. Infant's eyes irradiated unnecessarily.

Clinical equipment

Two ECG electrodes, nasogastric tube (NGT) and Replogle tube in situ.

Radiological interpretation

Mediastinum and heart normal. Lung fields normal. NGT tip and Replogle tube tip masked by overlying faciomaxillary structures (see above). Liver on the right. Stomach on the left. Gaseous distension of stomach and first part of duodenum in otherwise gasless abdomen.

Conclusion

Duodenal atresia in a preterm infant who was also found to have oesophageal atresia with a fistulous connection between the tracheobronchial tree and the lower oesophageal pouch. Neither NGT nor Replogle tube inserted sufficiently.

Suggest inserting the Replogle tube further, continuous aspiration and re-x-ray to check correct positioning of tip of Replogle tube.

CONGENITAL DIAPHRAGMATIC HERNIA

Frequency

1:4000 births

Pathology

▪ Persistence of foramen of Bochdalek (pleuroperitoneal canal) posterolaterally or foramen of Morgagni retrosternally.

▪ 90% are on the left side through the foramen of Bochdalek, and may contain small bowel, transverse colon, spleen and stomach.

▪ The associated pulmonary hypoplasia causes hypoxia and acidosis which lead to persistent fetal circulation syndrome.

▪ Occasionally associated volvulus of stomach.

▪ Frequently associated malrotation of midgut.

Presentation

▪ Respiratory distress at birth, the severity of which depends upon the size of the hernia.

▪ Ipsilateral chest is dull to percussion and may contain bowel sounds.

▪ Displacement of heart and mediastinum towards contralateral side.

▪ Scaphoid (relatively empty) abdomen.

Note

▪ **Bag and mask resuscitation contraindicated as bowel gaseous distension exacerbates respiratory symptoms and may be fatal.**

▪ **Pneumothoraces are a common complication.**

▪ **A nasogastric tube should be inserted and left on open drainage.**

▪ **Urgent transfer to a neonatal surgical unit is required.**

Differential diagnosis

- Congenital cystic adenomatoid malformations which are more common on the right and present later.

- Eventration (weakness) and paralysis of the diaphragm; the movement is paradoxical in the latter.

The radiographic features of congenital diaphragmatic hernia are illustrated in the following case studies.

CASE STUDY 53: AP VIEW OF CHEST AND UPPER ABDOMEN OF TERM INFANT

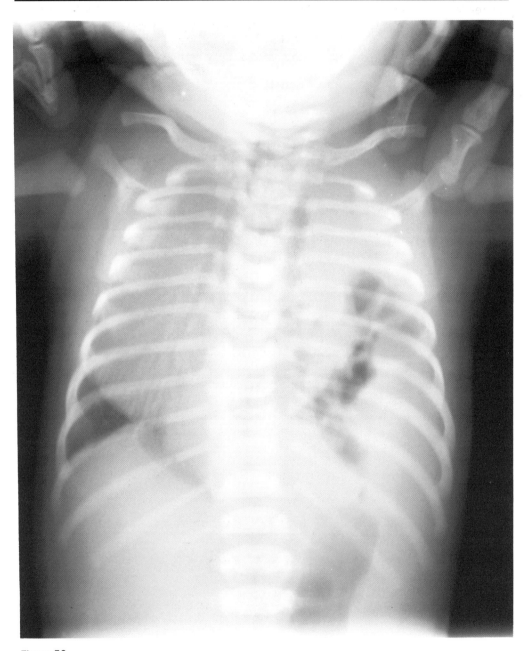

Figure 58

Technical comments

Exposure satisfactory (spine visible through heart shadow); inspiratory film (9 posterior rib ends above right diaphragm); rotated to the left (asymmetry of rib cage); mildly lordotic (upper ribs horizontal); head facing forwards. Assistant's fingers should not have been included in the field of exposure. Motional blurring of lung detail due to long exposure time of 0.04 s. (? inadequate mobile x-ray machine; see page 3).

Clinical equipment

Nil.

Radiological interpretation

Gross displacement of mediastinum and heart into the right chest by opaque left chest contents which show some aeration of bowel loops. Scaphoid abdomen. Liver in the right abdomen. No skeletal abnormalities.

Conclusion

Large left congenital diaphragmatic hernia in a term infant.
   Suggest immediate insertion of nasogastric tube on open drainage and appropriate management of respiratory distress.

Note

   An early film may show no bowel gas and complete opacification of hemithorax.

   Persistent fetal circulation and pneumothoraces are common complications.

CASE STUDY 54: AP VIEWS OF CHEST OF TERM INFANT

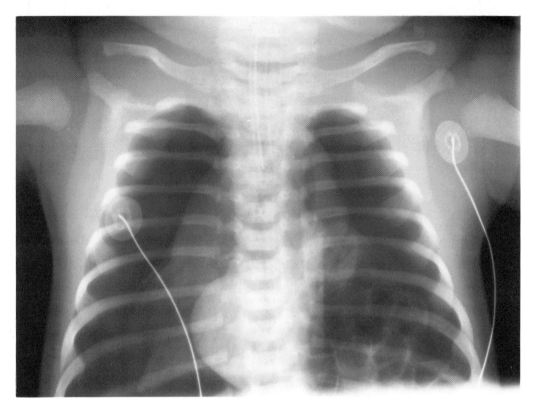

Figure 59a

Technical comments

Exposure satisfactory (spine visible through the heart shadow); overexpanded (10 posterior rib ends visible above right diaphragm); Figure 59a not rotated (anterior rib ends symmetrically placed), Figure 59b rotated to the left (asymmetry of rib cage); Figure 59a slightly lordotic (upper ribs horizontal), Figure 59b not lordotic (upper ribs appear to curve forwards and downwards); Figure 59a and b field size too restricted – should have included diaphragms and upper half of abdomen.

Clinical equipment

Figure 59a – Two ECG electrodes and an endotracheal tube (ETT) in situ.

Figure 59b – Two ECG electrodes, an endotracheal tube (ETT), a nasogastric tube (NGT) a right chest drain and a left chest butterfly needle drain in situ.

Radiological interpretation

Figure 59a – Massive bilateral pneumothoraces and loops of bowel in lower left chest. ETT tip at T3.

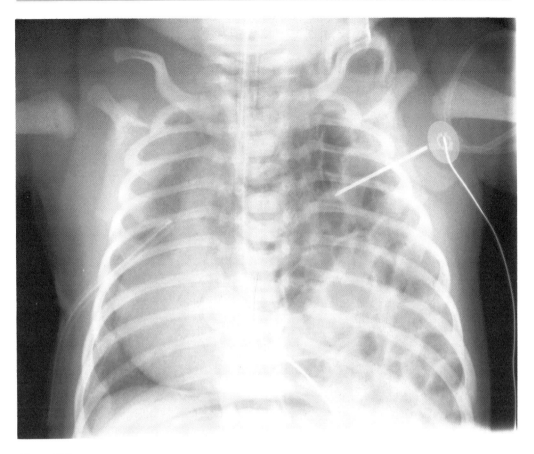

Figure 59b

Figure 59b – Mediastinum and heart grossly displaced into right chest by aerated loops of bowel in left chest. ETT tip at T2. Chest drains in situ as above. NGT passing into abdomen – tip not on film. Air under the diaphragm.

Conclusion

Bilateral massive pneumothoraces which have been drained, pneumoperitoneum and a large left congenital diaphragmatic hernia in a term infant on intensive care.
  Suggest:

1. Right lateral view of chest in the dorsal decubitus position (i.e. lying supine) with a horizontal x-ray beam to show possible anterior pneumothorax and position of chest drain tip.

2. AP view of abdomen with infant in supine position and vertical beam projection to identify gut obstruction.

3. AP view of abdomen with infant in left lateral decubitus position (right side up) and horizontal beam projection to confirm pneumoperitoneum and identify fluid levels of gut obstruction.

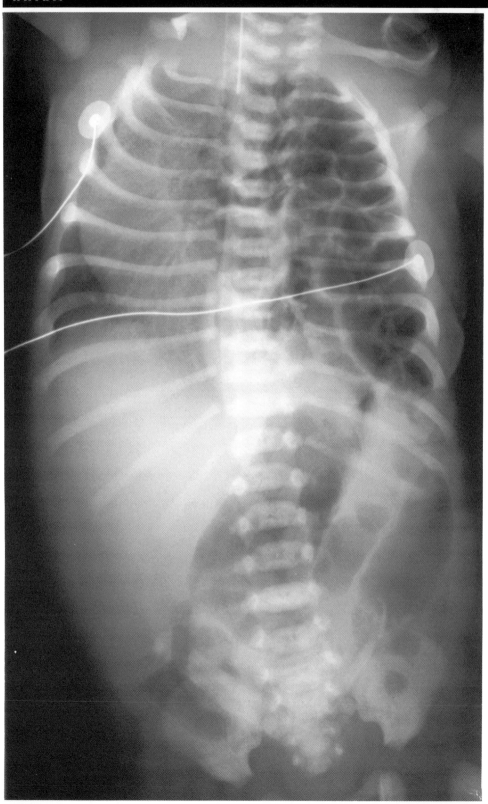

Figure 60

Technical comments

Slightly overexposed. Grossly rotated to the right (marked asymmetry of rib cage); marked lordosis (upper ribs appear to curve forwards and upwards). This infant has been x-rayed with no attempt at correct positioning.

Clinical equipment

Two ECG electrodes, endotracheal tube (ETT) and two transcutaneous blood gas monitor probe/sensor bases in situ.

Radiological interpretation

Left chest full of aerated loops of bowel causing deviation of heart and mediastinum to the right. ETT tip at T2. Liver under right hemidiaphragm. Central and left abdominal distended loops of bowel which are proximal to the bowel in the left chest.

Conclusion

Large left congenital diaphragmatic hernia and partially obstructed bowel in a term infant.
  Suggest immediate insertion of nasogastric tube on open drainage.

Note

▪ Possibility of volvulus of malrotated mid-gut loop should be considered.

CASE STUDY 56: AP VIEW OF PRETERM CHEST AND UPPER ABDOMEN

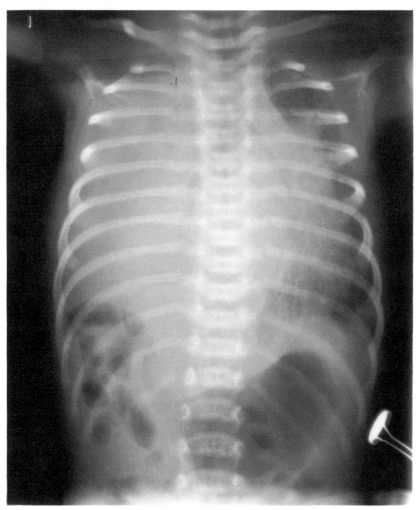

Figure 61

Technical comments

Exposure satisfactory (spine visible through heart shadow and left lung detail visible); overinflated (10 posterior rib ends visible above left diaphragm); rotated to the right (anterior rib ends asymmetrically placed and posterior ribs appear longer on right); lordotic (upper ribs are horizontal).

Clinical equipment

Single skin probe/sensor in situ.

Radiological interpretation

Mediastinum and heart displaced to the left. Complete homogeneous opacification of right chest. Left hemidiaphragm clearly seen. Right hemidiaphragm not seen. Bowel gas shadows seen immediately below where right hemidiaphragm would normally be expected. Gaseous distension of stomach.

Conclusion

Possible right congenital diaphragmatic hernia in a preterm infant.
   Suggest:

1. Immediate insertion of nasogastric tube on free drainage.

2. Repeat x-ray of chest and upper abdomen after interval of 30 minutes to identify whether there are bowel gas shadows in right chest.

CASE STUDY 57: AP VIEW OF FULL TERM CHEST AND UPPER ABDOMEN

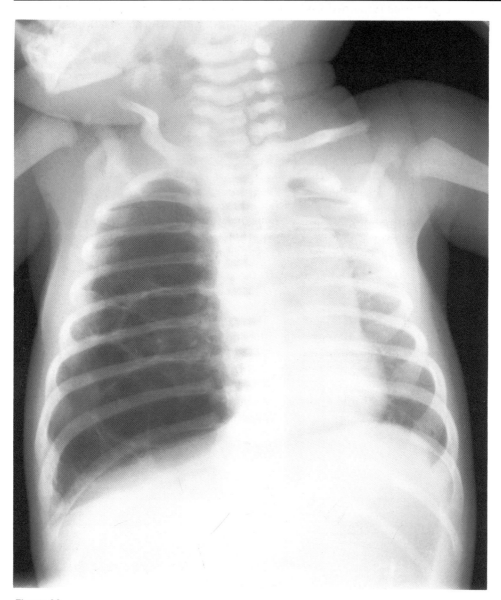

Figure 62

Technical comments

Exposure satisfactory (spine just visible through heart shadow); satisfactory inflation (9 posterior rib ends visible above right and left diaphragms); marked rotation to the right (anterior rib ends asymmetrically placed and posterior ribs appear longer on the right); not lordotic (upper ribs appear to curve forwards and downwards); head facing right.

Clinical equipment

Nil.

Radiological interpretation

Displacement of mediastinum and heart to the left. Loculated translucencies in right middle and lower lung fields with flattened right diaphragm. Increased density of left lung field due to compression collapse of left lung. No gas in upper abdomen.

Conclusion

Congenital cystic adenomatoid malformation of right lung.
 Differential diagnosis – right diaphragmatic hernia.

MEDIASTINAL MASSES

Chest masses do not present as emergencies unless they haemorrhage, become infected or compress adjacent vital structures. They may originate from the chest wall, lungs or mediastinum. The latter are most common and are classified according to their original location, i.e. anterior, middle or posterior mediastinum.

Anterior

- Thymus
- Thyroid
- Cystic hygroma
- Dermoid
- Teratoma.

Middle

- Bronchogenic cyst
- Duplication cyst.

Posterior

- Neuroblastoma
- Neurenteric cyst (may be associated with hemivertebra at T3)
- Intrathoracic meningocele.

CASE STUDY 58: AP VIEW OF CHEST OF INFANT

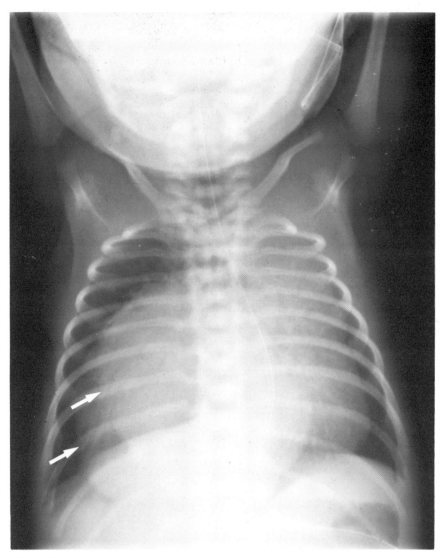

Figure 63

Technical comments

Exposure satisfactory (spine visible through heart shadow); inspiratory film (9 posterior rib ends visible above right diaphragm); not rotated (anterior rib ends symmetrically placed); not lordotic (upper ribs curve forwards and downwards); head facing forwards. Head should have been collimated out of x-ray field; arms need not have been raised.

Clinical equipment

Nasogastric tube (NGT) in situ.

Radiological interpretation

Heart, mediastinum and oesophagus (see course of NGT) displaced to the left by a large globular mass arising from middle and lower mediastinum and extending into right more than left chest. This homogeneous globular mass has a double right-sided margin (arrows) suggestive of a loculated cystic lesion. Abnormal upper thoracic vertebral bodies are present but with no rib abnormalities – erosions. Normal appearance to limited lung fields visible. Diaphragms intact. Liver on the right. NGT tip in stomach on the left.

Conclusion

Posterior mediastinal cystic mass associated with vertebral abnormalities suggestive of a neurenteric cyst. Needs to be differentiated from bronchogenic cyst.
    Suggest lateral view of chest to confirm posterior mediastinal location.

Note

▪ Posterior mediastinal calcification suggestive of neuroblastoma, whereas anterior mediastinal calcification suggestive of dermoid or teratoma.

The Abdomen

At birth in the term infant, swallowed air passes into the stomach and has reached the duodenum by 30–60 minutes, the jejunum by 2–4 hours, the ileum by 4–6 hours, the colon by 12–18 hours and the rectum by 24 hours, by which time more than 90% of newborns will have passed meconium. Gas in the rectum is an important radiological sign and usually indicates initial patency of the gastrointestinal tract, though subsequently the bowel may become obstructed, e.g. volvulus.

Note: gas may be introduced to the rectum by a thermometer or clinician's finger.

Normal radiological appearance of abdomen

■ Liver on the right; stomach on the left.

■ Marked variation in bowel gas patterns possible.

■ In general, loculated gas throughout small and large bowel to the rectum, with no prominent focal areas of bowel distension and fluid levels.

■ No evidence of free gas in peritoneum – must be excluded on every abdominal film; see p. 154 for radiological signs.

Decreased bowel gas	Increased bowel gas
Prolonged nasogastric aspiration	Delay in passage of meconium
Repeated vomiting	Respiratory distress
Conditions causing decreased	Paralytic ileus
swallowing/gut motility (e.g. prematurity)	Oesophageal atresia and fistula [*]
Paralysis with mechanical ventilation	Characteristic of H-type fistula [*]
Oesophageal atresia without fistula [*]	Mechanical obstruction of small or large bowel

[*] See section on oesophageal atresia.

Clinical presentation of pathology

■ Vomiting, which may be bile stained if obstruction is post ampullary.

■ Abdominal distension – absent in high obstructions.

■ Failure to pass meconium.

⬜ Blood-stained loose motions.

⬜ Signs of circulatory failure/sepsis neonatorum.

Alerting conditions

⬜ Omphaloceles and diaphragmatic hernia are associated with malrotation.

⬜ Down's syndrome and oesophageal atresia are associated with duodenal atresia.

⬜ Polyhydramnios is associated with oesophageal atresia and duodenal atresia.

Gastrointestinal tract pathology

Pathology	Figures	Radiological features
Paralytic ileus		Gaseous distension throughout small and large bowel with gas in rectum. No focal distended loops. Multiple long fluid levels (long because bowel flaccid) on gravity dependent views
Mechanical obstruction ⬜ Duodenal atresia/ stenosis/web ⬜ Annular pancreas	74–78	Double bubble appearance. Associated malrotation is common

⬜ Jejunal atresia/stenosis
⬜ Ileal atresia/stenosis
⬜ Malrotation ± volvulus
	79
	80–82
	85
		High obstruction – early presentation
		  – little abdominal distension
		Low obstruction – later presentation
		  – greater abdominal distension
		Focal loops of distended bowel stacked to give a step-ladder appearance (see Figure 85). Multiple short fluid levels (short because bowel peristalses) in proximal distended loops on gravity dependent views. No gas in rectum with congenital obstruction.

⬜ Meconium ileus *	83–84	Gaseous distension of small bowel and frothy appearance due to gas–meconium mix in right lower abdomen with no gas in rectum. Multiple small bowel fluid levels not always present on gravity dependent views. Associated small bowel atresia is common
⬜ Meconium plug syndrome ⬜ Hirschsprung's disease	100	Gaseous distension of small and large bowel to site of obstruction. No gas in rectum. Hirschsprung's may be complicated by necrotizing enterocolitis
⬜ Anorectal anomalies	101	See Case study 90
Necrotizing enterocolitis (NEC)	86–91 93–95 97–99	Abdominal distension, gaseous distension of small and large bowel, pneumatosis intestinalis (intramural gas) most often affecting caecal area, gas in the hepatic portal veins, perforation and pneumoperitoneum, ascites. **The translucency of the properitoneal fat line should not be confused with pneumatosis intestinalis** (see Figure 76).

* Stippled or curvilinear peritoneal calcification indicates antenatal bowel perforation and chemical peritonitis. Other causes of intra-abdominal calcification are adrenal (most common), renal, neuroblastoma, dermoids, teratoma and fetus in fetu.

Abdominal distension

There are many causes of abdominal distension. The infant's exact age, and history and the results of other investigations (e.g. ultrasound) need to be considered together to make a definitive diagnosis. For example, an early film or a paralysed infant's film showing a comparatively gasless abdomen may be misinterpreted as high gut obstruction; if taken before 24 hours of age for anorectal malformation the film will give a very misleading idea of the level of obstruction.

Bowel obstruction

As will be seen in the following films, **the diagnosis of gut obstruction can usually be made from the standard AP supine view**. If there is doubt, a horizontal beam AP view of the infant in the lateral decubitus position, which is a gravity-dependent view, will demonstrate the presence of fluid levels.

Bowel perforation

Gross pneumoperitoneum is radiologically obvious and is illustrated in the following case studies. However, **small amounts of free gas in the peritoneal cavity are most sensitively detected on a lateral view of the abdomen with the neonate in the dorsal decubitus (supine) position and a horizontal beam projection – a cross-table lateral view** (Figure 64).

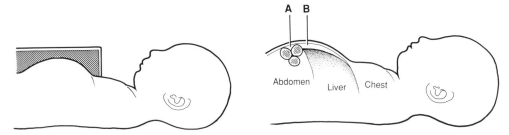

Figure 64. *Horizontal x-ray beam projection (cross-table lateral view).*

Small amounts of free gas may be seen as translucent inverted triangles (A) between adjacent loops of bowel and the peritoneal reflection on the anterior abdominal wall, or a translucent rim between the anterior surface of the liver and the anterior abdominal wall (B). An alternative method, though less sensitive and which involves handling/moving the sick neonate, is the AP view of the abdomen with the neonate in the left lateral decubitus (right side up) position and a horizontal beam projection (Figure 65).

This view again shows the translucencies of inverted triangles (A) between adjacent loops of bowel and the peritoneal reflection on the lateral abdominal wall, or a translucent rim between the lateral surface of the liver and the lateral abdominal wall.

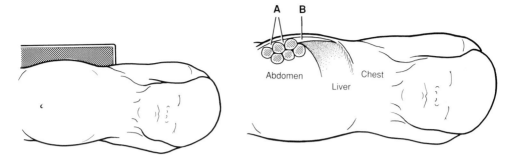

Figure 65. *Horizontal x-ray beam projection (cross-table AP view).*

Rarely, translucent triangles may be seen on a standard AP supine abdomen film (Figure 99). **Erect films involve excessive handling of the sick neonate and should NOT be requested.**

Note

■ For gut obstruction, the standard AP supine view can be supplemented by view A (see Figure 67) (which may show intraperitonal gas).

■ For necrotizing enterocolitis the standard AP supine view should be supplemented at regular intervals by view B (see Figure 68) to check for intraperitoneal gas.

Technical notes

Standard view: anteroposterior (AP) view with vertical beam, supine position (Figure 66)

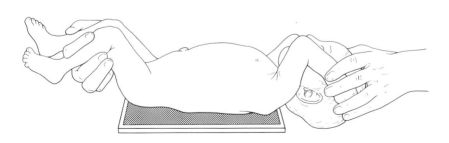

Figure 66

Common faults mostly concern inaccurate collimation of x-ray beam:

1. X-ray field too large, chest and legs irradiated unnecessarily

2. X-ray field too small:

   (a) diaphragm not included;

   (b) lateral collimation as for adults is not correct for neonates; it should be to the widest part of the abdomen.

The cassette should not be reversed to bring the name space to the bottom edge of film, as is the practice with adults. Very often it will obscure part of the lower gut or pelvis which may be diagnostically important (e.g. gas in rectum) (see Figure 76). Name space should be **outside** x-ray field.

Supplementary views

AP or PA view with horizontal beam, lateral decubitus position (Figure 67)

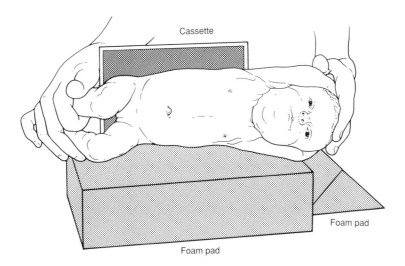

Cassette

Foam pad

Foam pad

Figure 67

This view is to show air–fluid levels in suspected bowel obstruction. The infant is laid on his or her side on a rectangular foam pad, to raise him or her above level of the incubator tray edge; arms are held raised by head, and hips (but not knees) extended. Infant's back must be touching cassette from shoulders to buttocks; he or she must not roll forwards.

Lateral view with horizontal beam, dorsal decubitus position (Figure 68)

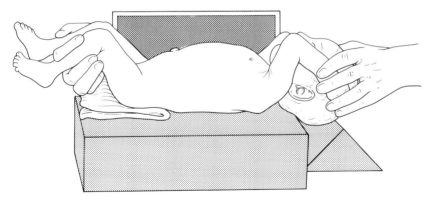

Figure 68

This view is the most sensitive radiographic technique for showing free air in the peritoneum after bowel perforation. The infant is laid on the back (foam pad not needed), arms held raised by head, legs extended (see Figure 91). *Note:* Exposure factors **less** than for AP view: anterior abdominal wall must be clearly seen.

Although the previously-described view (horizontal beam AP) is often taken to demonstrate free air, this lateral view is not only more sensitive but also entails far less handling of a fragile infant.

Lateral view with horizontal beam, prone position

For suspected 'imperforate anus' (anorectal anomalies) it has been traditional to take an inverted lateral view (baby held upside-down). The same information is gained by prone positioning with buttocks elevated on a 45° foam pad in the incubator (Figure 69). Less handling is involved, the infant is kept warm and can be left in position for the required 2–5 minutes before being x-rayed.

Exposure factors same as for AP view.

Cassette

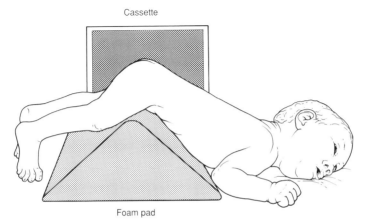

Foam pad

Figure 69

CASE STUDY 59: AP VIEW OF ABDOMEN OF TERM INFANT IN SUPINE POSITION WITH VERTICAL BEAM PROJECTION

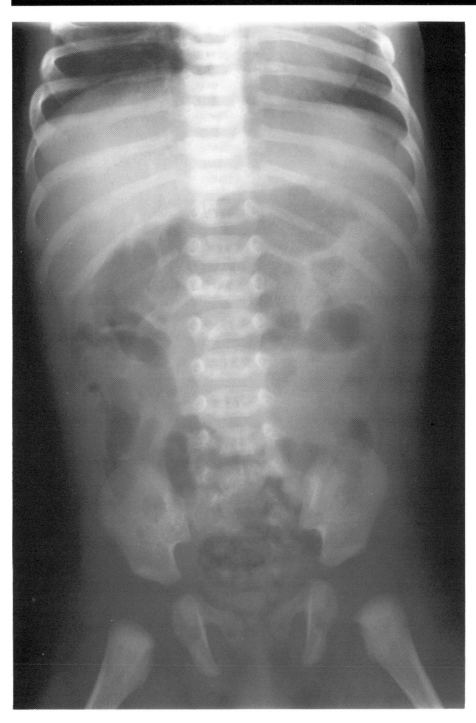

Figure 70

Technical comments

Exposure, positioning and collimation satisfactory.

Clinical equipment

Nil.

Radiological interpretation

Liver on the right. Stomach on the left. Loculated bowel gas shadows, in which no one loop stands out, extending into pelvic area. Gas/stool masses present in ascending and descending colon. Ribs, vertebral column, pelvis and upper femora appear normal.

Conclusion

Apparently normal abdomen of a term infant.

Note

- Normal term infants have gas throughout the bowel by 18–24 hours.
- Delay in the passage of bowel gas may occur in premature, sick or paralysed infants.
- The abdomen will be gasless below an oesophageal atresia without a fistula or an intestinal atresia.

CASE STUDY 60: AP VIEW OF ABDOMEN OF PRETERM INFANT IN SUPINE POSITION WITH VERTICAL BEAM PROJECTION

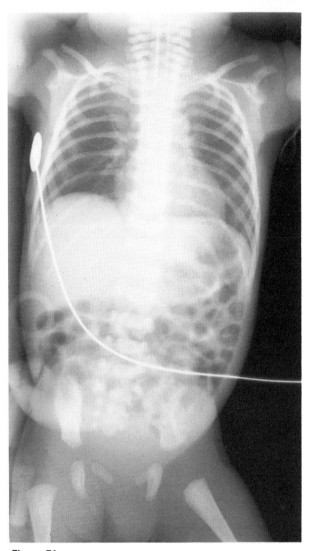

Figure 71

Technical comments

Exposure satisfactory. Abdomen rotated to the left (see iliac pelvis). The ECG lead should have been removed from field of interest.

Clinical equipment

ECG electrode and umbilical cord clamp in situ.

Radiological interpretation

Diaphragms intact. Liver on the right. Stomach on the left. Bowel gas shadows throughout abdomen but no gas in rectum.

Conclusion

Normal appearance to abdomen of markedly preterm infant but this interpretation (re rectal gas) is gestation and age dependent (see page 152).

CASE STUDY 61: LEFT LATERAL VIEW OF ABDOMEN AND LOWER CHEST OF TERM INFANT IN DORSAL DECUBITUS POSITION WITH HORIZONTAL BEAM PROJECTION

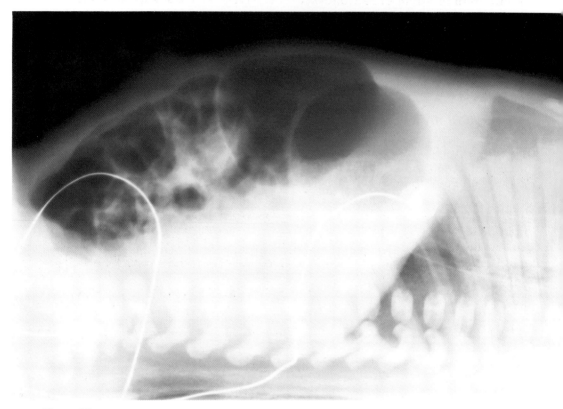

Figure 72

Technical comments

Good exposure (anterior abdominal wall clearly visible); not rotated (anterior rib ends coincide).

A common mistake of radiographers is to increase the exposure for lateral views (as for adults) which overexposes the anterior abdominal wall and thereby makes it invisible. Correct exposure is LESS than for the AP view.

Clinical equipment

Two ECG electrodes and a nasogastric tube (NGT) in situ.

Radiological interpretation

NGT tip in stomach. Gaseous distension of stomach and duodenum with normal loculated bowel gas shadows. No evidence of intramural gas or free gas in peritoneum, i.e. no gas triangles between loops of bowel and anterior abdominal wall or gas between surface of liver and anterior abdominal wall (see Figures 64, 93 and 94).

Conclusion

Normal appearance in a term infant.

CASE STUDY 62 (A SERIES OF TWO FILMS): AP VIEW OF CHEST AND ABDOMEN OF PRETERM INFANT IN SUPINE POSITION WITH VERTICAL BEAM PROJECTION

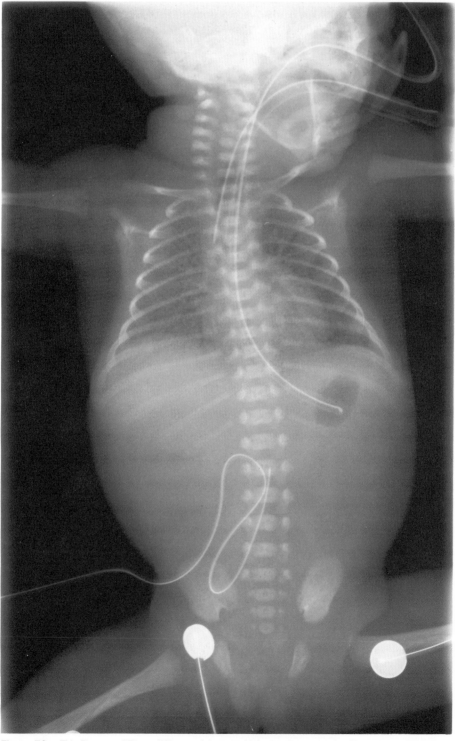

Figure 73a *This Figure and Figure 73b are of the same infant and consecutive films*

Technical comments

Figure 73a – Exposure satisfactory (spine visible through heart shadow); partial inspiration but acceptable (8 posterior rib ends visible above right diaphragm); no significant rotation (anterior rib ends symmetrically placed); not lordotic (upper ribs appear to curve forwards and downwards); field size too large, eyes irradiated unnecessarily.

Clinical equipment

Figure 73a – Two skin probes, endotracheal tube (ETT), nasogastric tube (NGT) umbilical arterial catheter (UAC) in situ.

Radiological interpretation

Figure 73a – Mediastinal and heart shadow appear normal. ETT tip at T3. Normal air bronchogram visible over cardiac shadow. Lung fields appear normal. Small gas shadow in stomach on the left. No other gas shadows in abdomen. NGT tip in stomach. UAC tip at L2 (renal artery level).

Conclusion

See p. 167.

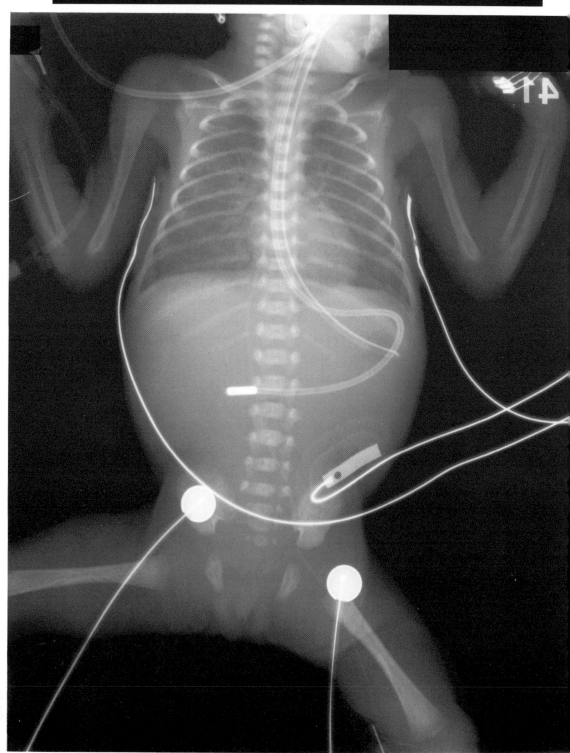

Figure 73b

Technical comments

Figure 73b – Exposure satisfactory (spine visible through heart shadow); inspiratory film (9 posterior rib ends visible above the right diaphragm); no significant rotation (anterior rib ends symmetrically placed); not lordotic (upper ribs appear to curve forwards and downwards); field size too large, gonads irradiated unnecessarily – arms and legs should have been excluded from x-ray field.

Clinical equipment

Figure 73b – Three ECG electrodes, two skin probes, endotracheal tube (ETT), nasogastric tube (NGT), nasojejunal tube (NJT) and left leg central venous line (CVL) in situ.

Radiological interpretation

Figure 73b – Mediastinal and heart shadow appear normal. ETT tip at T3. Horizontal fissure visible in right lung field. Lung fields appear normal. Small gas shadow in stomach on the left. No other gas shadows in abdomen. NGT tip in stomach. NJT tip in first part of duodenum. CVL tip at T8.

Conclusion

No abnormalities of chest or abdomen in a preterm infant on intensive care. Suggest relocation of UAC tip to either T9 or L3–4.

Note

▨ Airless abdomen normal only if less than 1 hour of age.

▨ For other causes of airless abdomen, see table on page 152.

CASE STUDY 63: AP VIEW OF ABDOMEN OF PRETERM INFANT IN SUPINE POSITION WITH VERTICAL BEAM PROJECTION

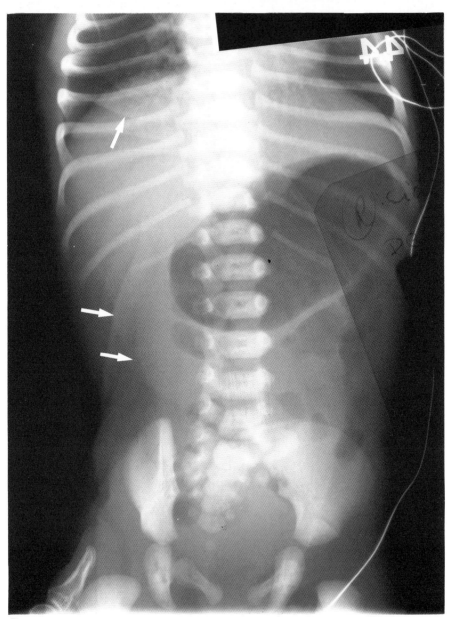

Figure 74

Technical comments

Exposure satisfactory. Lordotic and rotated view of lower chest gives right ribs their unusual appearance (rib 7 horizontal, 6 curves forwards and upwards). Spine curved and abdomen rotated to the left (note iliac pelvis). The positioning of this infant is unacceptable. Assistant's finger on right thigh should not have been included. Unacceptable superimposition of another radiograph over left abdomen.

Clinical equipment

Nasogastric tube (NGT) in situ.

Radiological interpretation

Diaphragms intact. Liver on the right. Stomach on the left. Gaseous distension of stomach but not duodenum. A number of small bowel gas shadows distal to pylorus. Prominent right abdominal skin creases (arrows).

Conclusion

Possible pyloric stenosis.
   Suggest ultrasound examination of pylorus.

CASE STUDY 64: AP VIEW OF ABDOMEN OF TERM INFANT IN SUPINE POSITION WITH VERTICAL BEAM PROJECTION

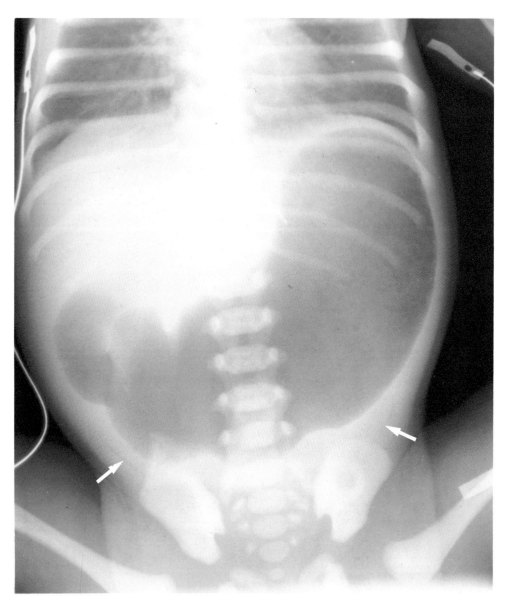

Figure 75

Technical comments

Underexposed film (too pale). Positioning and collimation satisfactory.

Clinical equipment

Three ECG electrodes and nasogastric tube (NGT) in situ.

Radiological interpretation

NGT tip in stomach. Gross gaseous distension of stomach and first part of duodenum giving double bubble appearance. No free gas in peritoneum (see pages 154–5). No bowel gas shadows in rest of abdomen. Diaphragms intact. Liver on the right. Stomach on the left. Pelvic bones not suggestive of Down's syndrome. Bilateral properitoneal fat lines just visible (arrows).

Conclusion

Duodenal obstruction in term infant.

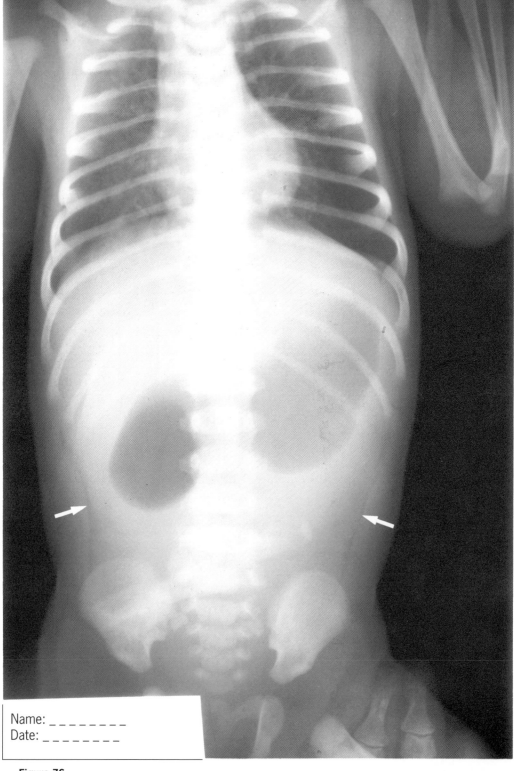

Name: _ _ _ _ _ _ _ _
Date: _ _ _ _ _ _ _ _

Figure 76

Technical comments

Exposure satisfactory for chest but slightly underexposed for abdomen – not achievable in a term infant because abdomen would require greater exposure than chest; expiratory film (7 posterior rib ends visible above right diaphragm); not significantly rotated (anterior rib ends symmetrically placed); lordotic view (upper ribs horizontal) because centring is on abdomen. Chest and left arm have been irradiated unnecessarily. The pelvis is partly obscured by the name space, which should appear at the top of the film outside the x-ray field (see page 156). Assistant's fingers on the left thigh should not have been included.

Clinical equipment

Nasogastric tube (NGT) and umbilical clamp in situ.

Radiological interpretation

Mediastinum and heart shadows normal. Despite expiration heart apex appears elevated off the left diaphragm because of lordotic view. Increased translucency of left lower lung field. Otherwise lung fields normal. Diaphragms normal. Liver on the right. Stomach on the left. Gas in stomach and first and second part of duodenum with no bowel gas distal to this. Pelvic bones not suggestive of Down's syndrome. Bilateral properitoneal fat lines clearly visible (arrows). Speckled dark artefact over left abdomen. NGT tip not visible.

Conclusion

Duodenal obstruction in a preterm infant.
   Suggest AP chest in the right lateral decubitus position (left side up) with a horizontal beam projection in order to exclude a small left pneumothorax.

CASE STUDY 66: AP VIEW OF ABDOMEN OF TERM INFANT IN LEFT LATERAL DECUBITUS POSITION WITH HORIZONTAL BEAM PROJECTION

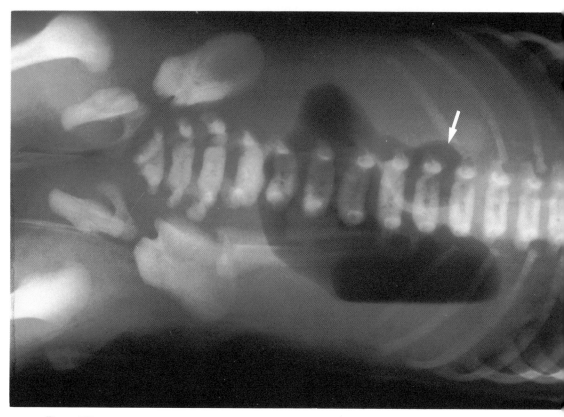

Figure 77

Technical comments

Slightly overexposed (dark film). (**Note: this is correct positioning, not the traditional erect position**.)

Clinical equipment

Plastic umbilical cord clamp in situ.

Radiological interpretation

Fluid level in stomach. Gaseous distension of stomach and first part of duodenum (arrow) giving double bubble appearance. No bowel gas shadows in rest of abdomen. No free gas in peritoneum. Diaphragms intact. Liver on the right. Stomach on the left. Pelvic bones not suggestive of Down's syndrome.

Conclusion

Duodenal obstruction in a term infant.

CASE STUDY 67: AP VIEW OF ABDOMEN AND CHEST OF PRETERM INFANT IN ERECT POSITION WITH A HORIZONTAL BEAM PROJECTION

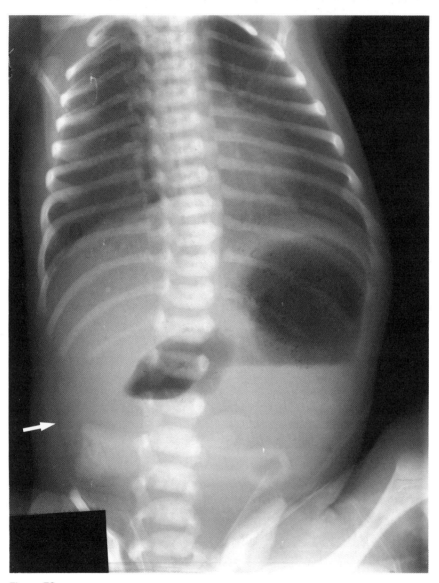

Figure 78

Technical comments

Traditional erect position is unnecessary to prove fluid levels in 'double bubble' sign: supporting infant and cassette erect poses great problems in special care baby unit. Same information is obtained with lateral decubitus positioning of infant in the incubator (see Figure 77) (Gyll, 1985). Exposure satisfactory (spine visible through heart shadow); part inspiratory film (8 posterior rib ends visible above the right diaphragm); rotated to the left (anterior rib ends asymmetrically placed and posterior ribs longer on the left); lordotic (upper ribs appear to curve forwards and upwards). Multiple photographic artefacts, and nappy folds over left lower abdomen.

Clinical equipment

Nasogastric tube (NGT) and plastic umbilical clamp in situ.

Radiological interpretation

No abnormalities of heart and lungs. Gaseous distension of stomach and first part of duodenum (double bubble appearance) which both contain a fluid level. No bowel gas in rest of abdomen. No free gas in peritoneal cavity under diaphragm. NGT in stomach. Diaphragms intact. Liver on the right. Stomach on the left. Right-sided properitoneal fat line visible (arrow).

Conclusion

Duodenal obstruction in a preterm infant.

CASE STUDY 68: AP VIEW OF CHEST AND ABDOMEN OF PRETERM INFANT IN SUPINE POSITION WITH VERTICAL BEAM PROJECTION

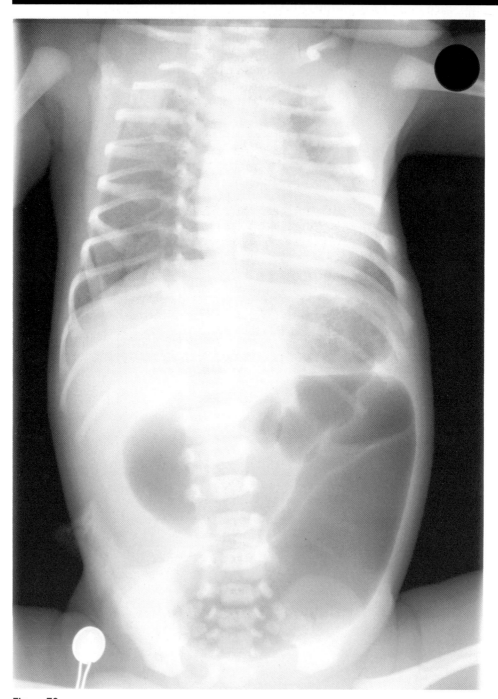

Figure 79

Technical comments

Exposure unsatisfactory (pale film); part inspiratory film (8 posterior rib ends visible above the right diaphragm); marked rotation to the left (rib cage asymmetrical); lordotic view (upper ribs horizontal) because centring is on abdomen. Chest has been irradiated unnecessarily; this distorted view is not diagnostic.

Clinical equipment

Umbilical cord clamp and skin probe in situ.

Radiological interpretation

Mediastinum and heart rotated to the left. Visible lung fields appear normal. Note prominent skin crease in right lower lung field. Diaphragms intact. Liver on the right. Stomach on the left. Gross gaseous distension of stomach, duodenum and jejunum with no bowel gas distal to this.

Conclusion

Jejunal obstruction – probable atresia (very rare) – in a preterm infant.

CASE STUDY 69: AP VIEW OF ABDOMEN, INCLUDING CHEST, OF A PRETERM INFANT IN SUPINE POSITION WITH VERTICAL BEAM PROJECTION

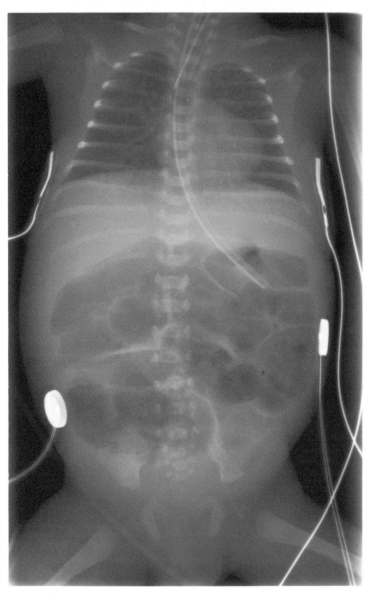

Figure 80

Technical comments

Exposure of abdomen satisfactory (good bowel gas shadow detail). Chest exposure unsatisfactory (too dark); expiratory film (7 posterior rib ends visible above right diaphragm) and markedly lordotic (ribs curve forwards and upwards) because centring has been on abdomen. Chest has been irradiated unnecessarily; this distorted view is not diagnostic.

Clinical equipment

Two ECG electrodes, two skin probes/sensors, an endotracheal tube (ETT), a nasogastric tube (NGT) and a left leg central venous line (CVL) in situ.

Radiological interpretation

Distended abdomen. Liver on the right. NGT tip in stomach on the left. Gaseous distension of multiple loops of bowel. No signs of intramural gas or intraperitoneal gas. No gas in rectum. ETT tip at T3. Heart shape and the appearance of apex of heart elevated off the diaphragm are probably due to lordotic view. Normal vascularity of lung fields not suggestive of Fallot's tetralogy. Position of CVL tip unclear.

Conclusion

Probable ileal obstruction in a preterm infant.
   Suggest:

1. If diagnosis of obstruction is in doubt, AP view of abdomen in left lateral decubitus position with a horizontal beam projection to show fluid levels.

2. Correctly exposed (see page 5) lateral view of abdomen in dorsal decubitus position with a horizontal beam to check if free air is present in the peritoneal cavity.

CASE STUDY 70: AP VIEW OF ABDOMEN OF PRETERM INFANT IN SUPINE POSITION WITH VERTICAL BEAM PROJECTION

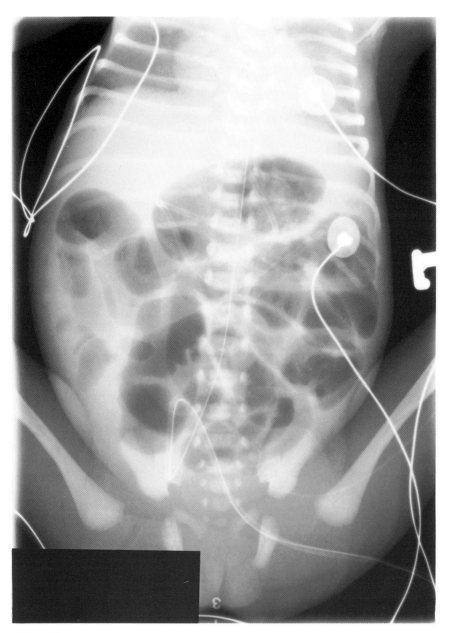

Figure 81

Technical comments

Exposure, positioning and collimation satisfactory.

Clinical equipment

Two ECG electrodes, nasogastric tube (NGT), umbilical arterial catheter (UAC) and left femoral central venous line (CVL) in situ.

Radiological interpretation

Diaphragms intact. Liver on the right. Stomach on the left. NGT tip obscured by overlying ECG electrode on left hypochondrium. Marked gaseous distension of loops of small bowel throughout abdomen. No gas in rectum. No radiological signs of intramural gas or free gas in peritoneal cavity. UAC tip at T8. CVL tip location unclear.

Conclusion

Probable small bowel obstruction in a preterm infant.
    Suggest:

1. AP view of abdomen in left lateral decubitus position with a horizontal beam projection to show fluid levels.

2. Correctly exposed (see page 5) lateral view of abdomen in dorsal decubitus position, with horizontal beam to show free air in peritoneal cavity.

CASE STUDY 71 (A SERIES OF TWO FILMS): AP VIEW OF CHEST AND ABDOMEN OF TERM INFANT IN SUPINE POSITION WITH VERTICAL BEAM PROJECTION

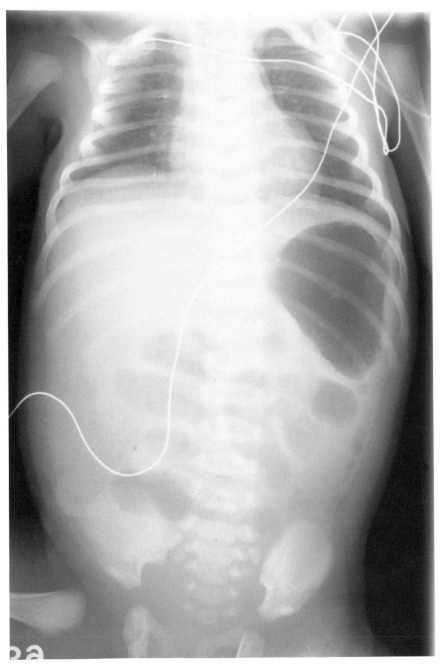

Figure 82a

Technical comments

Figure 82a – Exposure unsatisfactory for abdomen (too pale: abdomen requires greater exposure than chest in term infants); expiratory film (6 posterior ribs visible above right diaphragm); not rotated (anterior rib ends symmetrically placed); lordotic (upper ribs appear horizontal). Chest has been irradiated unnecessarily.

Clinical equipment

Figure 82a – ECG electrodes and leads and nasogastric tube (NGT) in situ.

Radiological interpretation

Figure 82a – Mediastinum, heart and lung fields appear normal. Abdominal distension causing chest compression. Diaphragms intact. Liver on the right. Stomach on the left. Gaseous distension of stomach and loops of bowel which are just visible in centre of abdomen. Possibly some gas in descending colon. No gas in rectum.

Conclusion

See p. 187.

CASE STUDY 71 (CONTINUED)**: AP VIEW OF ABDOMEN OF TERM INFANT IN LEFT LATERAL DECUBITUS POSITION WITH HORIZONTAL BEAM PROJECTION**

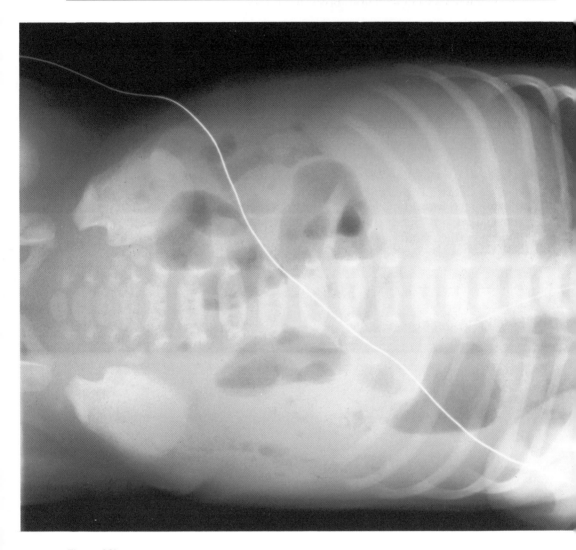

Figure 82b

Technical comments

Figure 82b – Exposure, positioning and collimation satisfactory. ECG lead should have been moved from field of interest, in both films.

Clinical equipment

Figure 82b – ECG lead and nasogastric tube (NGT) in situ.

Radiological interpretation

Figure 82b – Air–fluid level in stomach, and multiple air–fluid levels in small bowel. No free gas in peritoneal cavity around right lower liver edge. Horizontal line artefact over left abdomen is probably due to edge of incubator tray.

Conclusion

Incomplete ileal obstruction in term infant.

CASE STUDY 72: AP VIEW OF ABDOMEN OF INFANT IN ERECT POSITION WITH HORIZONTAL BEAM PROJECTION

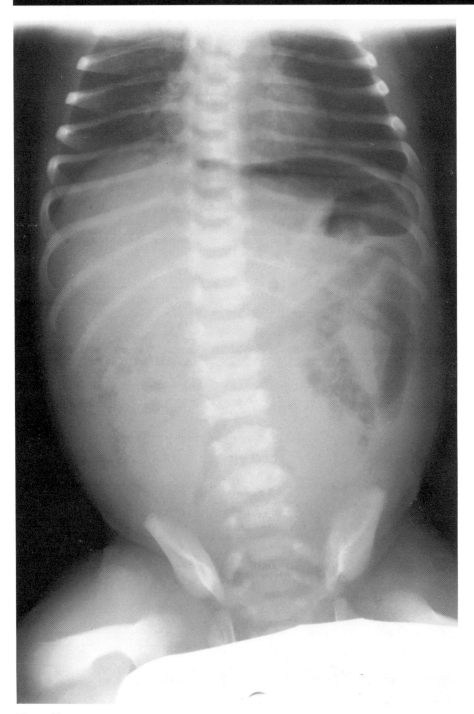

Figure 83

Technical comment

Exposure satisfactory. **Erect position is unnecessary to prove free gas or fluid levels: supporting infant and cassette erect poses great problems in a special care baby unit. Same information is obtained with lateral** (see Figure 77) **or dorsal decubitus** (see Figures 93 and 94) **positioning of infant in incubator (has to be taken out for erect positioning).**

Clinical equipment

Nasogastric tube (NGT) in situ.

Radiological interpretation

Free gas in peritoneal cavity under left diaphragm. Liver on the right. NGT tip in stomach on the left. Gas/meconium 'bubbly' appearance in right lateral abdomen. Gaseous distension of small bowel proximal to terminal ileum with bubbly appearance to contents. No gas in colon. No gas–fluid levels visible: a sign highly suggestive of meconium ileus.

Conclusion

Meconium ileus leading to bowel perforation and gas in the peritoneal cavity.

CASE STUDY 73: AP VIEW OF ABDOMEN OF INFANT IN LEFT LATERAL DECUBITUS POSITION WITH HORIZONTAL BEAM PROJECTION

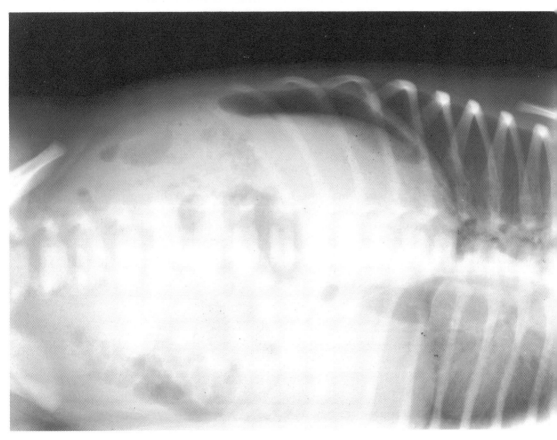

Figure 84

Technical comment

Exposure, positioning and collimation satisfactory.

Clinical equipment

Nasogastric tube in situ.

Radiological interpretation

Free gas in the peritoneal cavity under right diaphragm. Liver on the right. NGT tip in stomach on the left. Gaseous distension of two loops of small bowel in central abdomen. Gas/meconium 'bubbly' appearance in right and left abdomen. No gas–fluid levels visible: a sign suggestive of meconium ileus.

Conclusion

Meconium ileus leading to bowel perforation and gas in the peritoneal cavity.

Note

▪ Dorsal decubitus position is less disturbing for ill infant with suspected perforation (less handling).

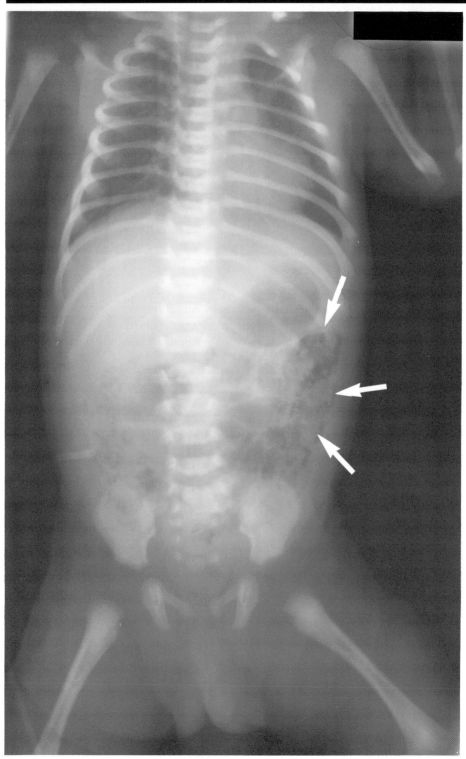

Figure 86a

Technical comments

Figure 86a – Exposure satisfactory for abdomen, chest overexposed; partial inspiratory film (8 posterior rib ends visible above right diaphragm); chest markedly rotated to the left (anterior rib ends asymmetrically placed and posterior ribs longer on the left) but abdomen not rotated (lower ribs and pelvis symmetrical); poor collimation: chest and limbs irradiated unnecessarily.

Clinical equipment

Figure 86a – Catheter shadow superimposed on right thigh and right lower abdomen – probably superfluous and if so it should have been removed.

Radiological interpretation

Figure 86a – Diaphragms intact. Liver on the right. Stomach on the left. Bowel gas shadows in central abdomen with distended ascending and descending colon containing stool–gas mixture; gas in walls of descending colon – pneumatosis intestinalis (arrows).

Conclusion

See p. 197

CASE STUDY 75 (CONTINUED): AP VIEW OF ABDOMEN OF PRETERM INFANT IN LEFT LATERAL DECUBITUS POSITION WITH HORIZONTAL BEAM PROJECTION

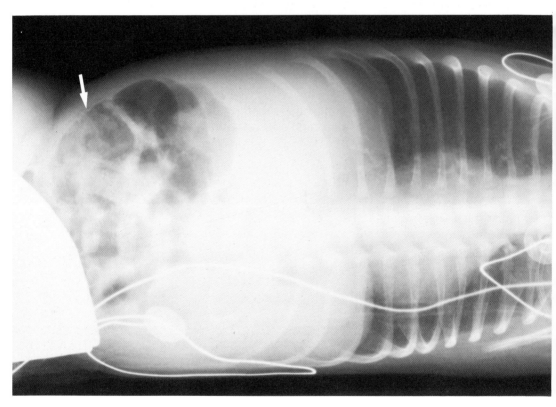

Figure 86b

Technical comments

Figure 86b – Exposure satisfactory. Chest should not have been included as satisfactory AP view of chest is not possible in this position. Chest irradiated unnecessarily. Gonad shield misplaced and obscuring part of abdomen.

Clinical equipment

Figure 86b – Three ECG electrodes/leads and nasogastric tube (NGT) in situ.

Radiological interpretation

Figure 86b – gaseous distension of loops of bowel in right lower abdomen with gas in wall of caecum (arrow); no free gas in peritoneal cavity (see Figure 65); rectum obscured by gonad shield.

Conclusion

Pneumatosis intestinalis suggestive of necrotizing enterocolitis in a preterm infant. No evidence of bowel perforation.

Suggest repeat films at regular intervals to exclude bowel perforation and free gas in the peritoneal cavity – lateral views of abdomen in dorsal decubitus position with horizontal beam projection (see page 157) and correct exposure (see page 5).

CASE STUDY 76: AP VIEW OF ABDOMEN OF INFANT IN SUPINE POSITION WITH VERTICAL BEAM PROJECTION

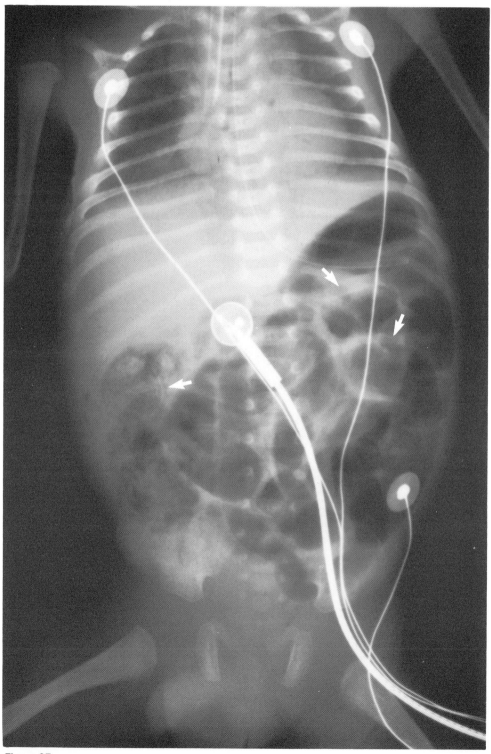

Figure 87

Technical comments

Exposure satisfactory for abdomen. Monitoring leads should have been removed from field of interest. Gonads irradiated. Poor collimation: x-ray field too large, chest irradiated unnecessarily.

Clinical equipment

Three ECG electrodes, monitoring skin probe/sensor, endotracheal tube (ETT) and nasogastric tube (NGT) in situ.

Radiological interpretation

Diaphragms indistinctly seen. Liver on the right. Stomach on the left. NGT tip in stomach. Bowel gas shadows throughout abdomen. Bowel wall thickening (arrows) in left upper quadrant. Hepatic flexure of colon seen end on with possibly some intramural gas giving double ring sign appearance (arrow). No gas in rectum. No radiological signs of gas in peritoneal cavity. ETT tip in right lower lobe bronchus. This expiratory lordotic view of chest is not diagnostic and may be misleading.

Conclusion

Signs of necrotizing enterocolitis in an infant on intensive care.
  Suggest:

1. ETT should be withdrawn immediately by 3 cm.

2. Chest x-ray to confirm or exclude lobar collapse.

3. Repeat films at regular intervals to exclude bowel perforation and gas in the peritoneal cavity – lateral views of abdomen in dorsal decubitus position with horizontal beam projection (see page 157) and correct exposure (see page 5).

CASE STUDY 77: AP VIEW OF ABDOMEN OF PRETERM INFANT IN SUPINE POSITION WITH VERTICAL BEAM PROJECTION

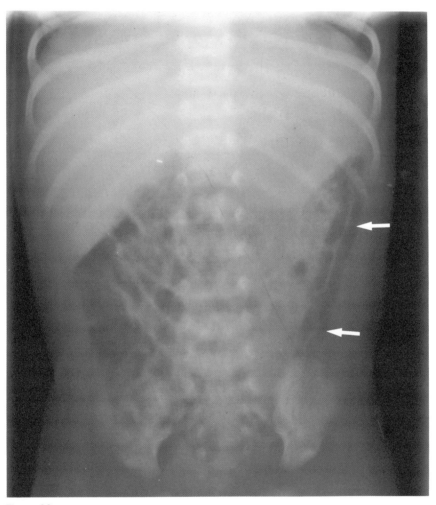

Figure 88

Technical comments

Exposure satisfactory. Diaphragms should have been included within x-ray field.

Clinical equipment

Nil.

Radiological interpretation

Liver on the right. Stomach on the left. Gas shadows throughout small and large bowel. Gaseous distension of ascending and descending colon. Gas in bowel wall – pneumatosis intestinalis (arrows) – of descending colon. No gas in rectum. Diaphragms not visualized. No free gas visible in peritoneal cavity.

Conclusion

Pneumatosis intestinalis suggestive of necrotizing enterocolitis in a preterm infant.

Suggest correctly exposed lateral view of abdomen in dorsal decubitus position with horizontal x-ray beam projection at regular intervals to exclude pneumoperitoneum (see pages 154–5).

CASE STUDY 78: AP VIEW OF ABDOMEN OF SLIGHTLY PRETERM INFANT IN SUPINE POSITION WITH VERTICAL BEAM PROJECTION

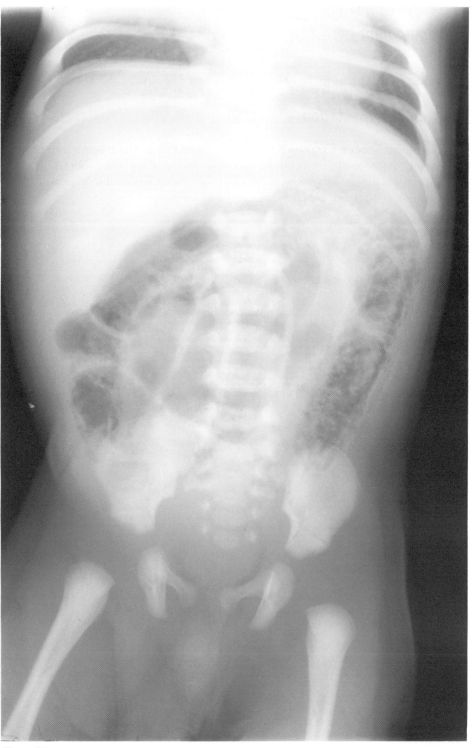

Figure 89

Technical comment

Slightly underexposed (film too pale). Gonads irradiated unnecessarily.

Clinical equipment

Nil.

Radiological interpretation

Diaphragm intact. Liver on the right. Stomach probably on the left. Dilated bowel gas shadows clearly seen in central abdomen and descending colon. Gross pneumatosis intestinalis (intramural gas) of ascending and descending colon. No gas in rectum.

Conclusion

Necrotizing enterocolitis of ascending and descending colon.

Suggest lateral view of abdomen in dorsal decubitus position (lying supine) with horizontal beam projection at regular intervals to exclude free gas in the peritoneal cavity.

CASE STUDY 79 (A SERIES OF TWO FILMS): AP VIEW OF CHEST AND ABDOMEN OF PRETERM INFANT IN SUPINE POSITION WITH VERTICAL BEAM PROJECTION

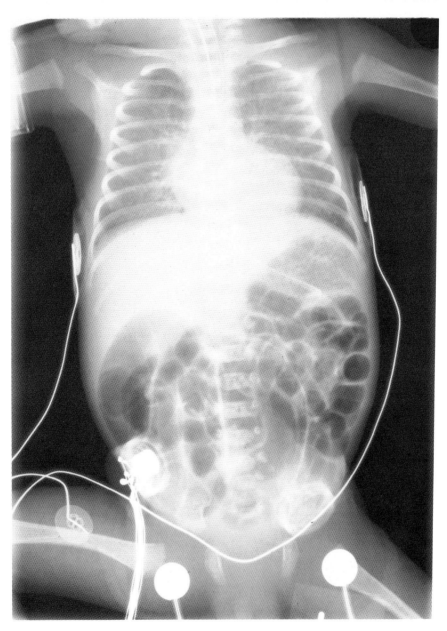

Figure 90a

Technical comments

Figure 90a – Slightly underexposed (spine barely visible through heart shadow); partial inspiration (8 posterior rib ends visible above the right diaphragm); not rotated (anterior rib ends symmetrically placed); lordotic view of chest because x-ray beam is centred to abdomen (see Figure 2).

Clinical equipment

Figure 90a – Three ECG electrodes, two skin probes/sensors, a transcutaneous blood gas monitor probe/sensor and separate base, an endotracheal tube (ETT) and a nasogastric tube (NGT) in situ.

Radiological interpretation

Figure 90a – Mediastinum and heart appear normal. ETT tip at T3–4. Lung field appearances compatible with hyaline membrane disease. NGT tip in stomach. Gas in stomach and throughout bowel. Distended loop of bowel under liver. No obvious bowel wall thickening or intramural gas. No characteristic triangles of free gas in peritoneal cavity and no gas in rectum.

Conclusion

Respiratory distress syndrome and no clear evidence of necrotizing enterocolitis or bowel perforation.

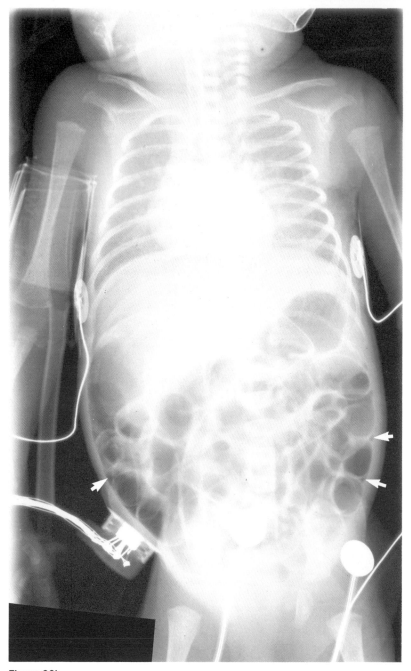

Figure 90b

Technical comments

Figure 90b – Slightly underexposed (spine barely visible through heart shadow); expiratory film (7 posterior rib ends visible above the right diaphragm); grossly rotated to the right (anterior rib ends asymmetrically placed and posterior ribs appear longer on the right); lordotic view of chest because x-ray beam is centred to abdomen (see Figure 2).

Clinical equipment

Figure 90b – Two ECG electrodes, two skin probes/sensors, a transcutaneous blood gas monitor probe/sensor, a blood pressure cuff, an endotracheal tube (ETT) and a nasogastric tube (NGT) in situ.

Radiological interpretation

Figure 90b – Mediastinum and heart rotated to the right. ETT tip at T3 at carina. Lung field appearances compatible with hyaline membrane disease. Abdominal appearances as above but now there are characteristic translucent triangles (arrows) in both flanks indicative of free gas in the peritoneal cavity. Also air under right diaphragm.

Conclusion

Respiratory distress syndrome and early bowel perforation probably due to necrotizing enterocolitis in a preterm infant on intensive care.
    Suggest ETT tip withdrawn by 1 cm.

CASE STUDY 80: AP VIEW OF ABDOMEN OF PRETERM INFANT IN LEFT LATERAL DECUBITUS POSITION WITH HORIZONTAL BEAM PROJECTION

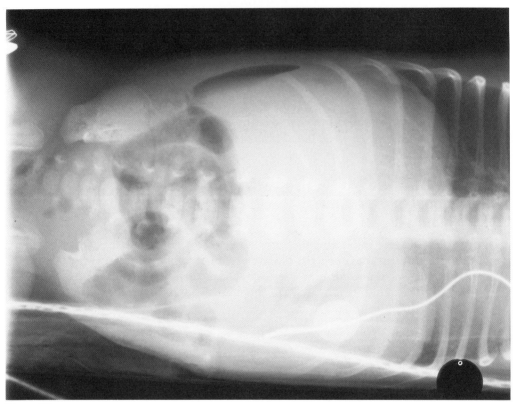

Figure 91

Technical comments

Exposure, positioning and collimation satisfactory. Monitoring equipment leads should have been removed from field of interest.

Clinical equipment

One ECG electrode, leads and nasogastric tube (NGT) in situ.

Radiological interpretation

Diaphragms intact. Liver on the right. Stomach on the left. Gaseous distension of loops of bowel in lower abdomen with gas in bowel wall in right iliac fossa. Free gas in peritoneal cavity.

Conclusion

Necrotizing enterocolitis causing intestinal perforation in a preterm infant.

Note

▓ A lateral abdomen view in the dorsal decubitus position with a horizontal beam projection (see Figure 68) would have been less disturbing (less handling) for the ill infant.

CASE STUDY 81: AP VIEW OF ABDOMEN OF INFANT IN RIGHT LATERAL DECUBITUS POSITION WITH HORIZONTAL BEAM PROJECTION

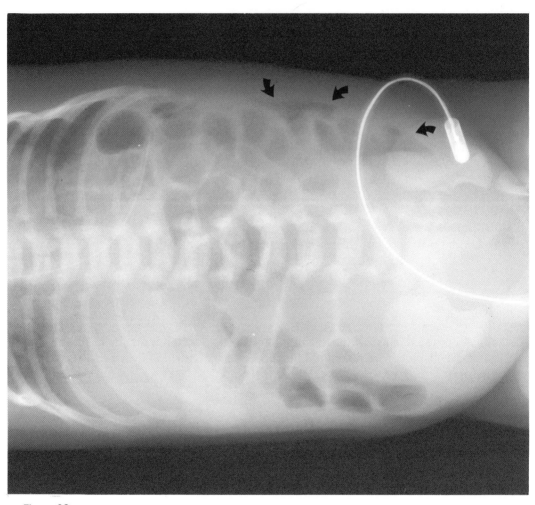

Figure 92

Technical comments

Exposure, positioning and collimation satisfactory.

Clinical equipment

Skin probe and nasogastric tube (NGT) in situ.

Radiological interpretation

Liver on the right. NGT tip in stomach on the left. Bowel gas shadows throughout abdomen. Characteristic triangular shadows (arrows) of free gas in peritoneal cavity in left flank, easily missed.

Conclusion

Free gas in peritoneal cavity probably due to bowel perforation.

Note

▪ A lateral abdomen view in the dorsal decubitus position with a horizontal beam projection would have been less disturbing (less handling) for the ill infant.

CASE STUDY 82: LATERAL VIEW OF ABDOMEN OF INFANT IN DORSAL DECUBITUS POSITION WITH HORIZONTAL BEAM PROJECTION

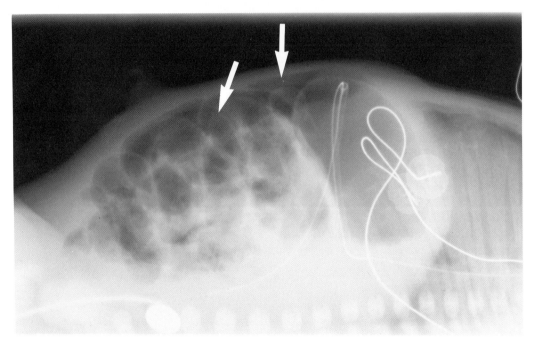

Figure 93

Technical comments

Exposure satisfactory (anterior abdominal wall visible); also positioning and collimation.

Clinical equipment

Two ECG electrodes, a skin probe/sensor and nasogastric tube (NGT) in situ.

Radiological interpretation

Characteristic triangles (arrow) of free gas in anterior peritoneal cavity. Intramural bowel gas (arrow). Gaseous distension of multiple loops of bowel. NGT passing through stomach with tip in second part of duodenum.

Conclusion

Bowel perforation due to necrotizing enterocolitis.
   Suggest withdrawal of NGT tip to stomach.

CASE STUDY 83: LATERAL VIEW OF ABDOMEN OF INFANT IN DORSAL DECUBITUS POSITION WITH HORIZONTAL BEAM PROJECTION

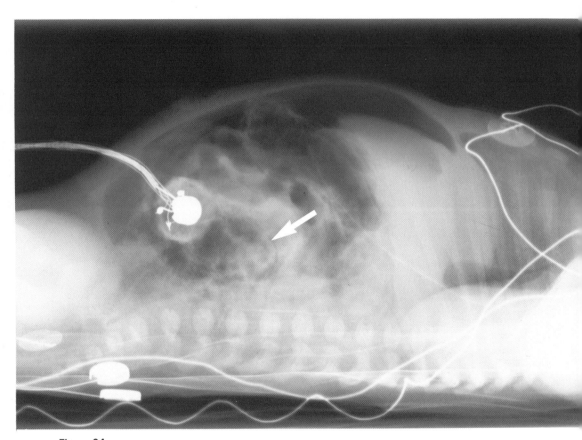

Figure 94

Technical comments

Exposure satisfactory (anterior abdominal wall visible); positioning and collimation satisfactory.

Clinical equipment

Three ECG electrodes, two other skin probes, a transcutaneous blood gas monitor probe/sensor and a nasogastric tube (NGT) in situ.

Radiological interpretation

Large collection of free gas in anterior peritoneal cavity. Air in the oesophagus. NGT tip in stomach. Intramural bowel gas (arrow).

Conclusion

Bowel perforation due to necrotizing enterocolitis.

CASE STUDY 84: AP VIEW OF ABDOMEN OF SLIGHTLY PRETERM INFANT IN ERECT POSITION WITH HORIZONTAL BEAM PROJECTION

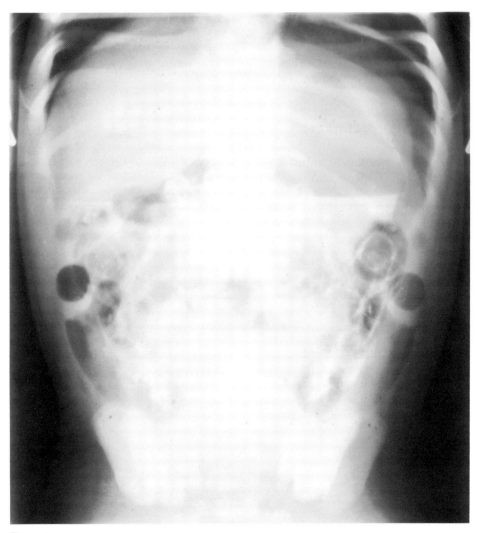

Figure 95

Technical comments

Erect positioning is condemned. Decubitus positioning must always be used. Exposure unsatisfactory (too pale). Poor collimation – right diaphragm not seen, particularly important in this case – see below.

Clinical equipment

None.

Radiological interpretation

Diaphragm clearly seen only on the left with large gas collection in the peritoneal cavity below it. Liver on the right. Stomach on the left. Both right and left abdomen show clear bowel gas shadows and gas-distended loops of bowel end on (ring sign). On the left one of these loops shows a double ring sign suggestive of gross intramural gas, i.e. pneumatosis intestinalis.

Conclusion

Gas in the peritoneal cavity due to perforated necrotizing enterocolitis.

CASE STUDY 85: AP VIEW OF CHEST AND ABDOMEN OF PRETERM INFANT IN SUPINE POSITION WITH VERTICAL BEAM PROJECTION

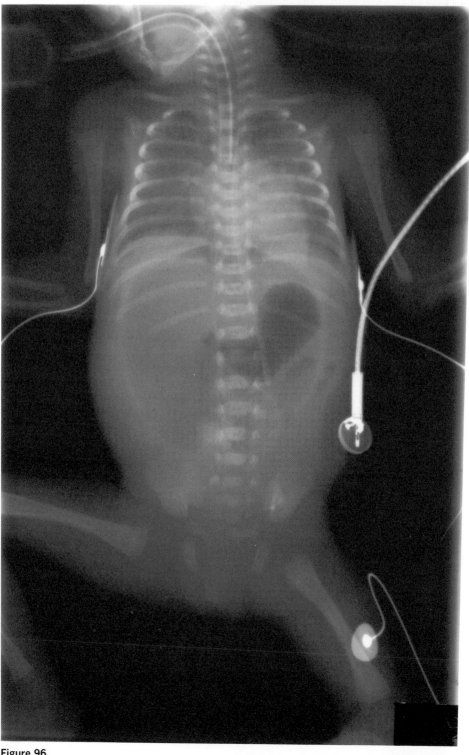

Figure 96

Technical comments

Exposure unsatisfactory for chest (too dark); just satisfactory for abdomen (also dark); expiratory film (7 posterior rib ends visible above the right diaphragm); not rotated (anterior rib ends symmetrically placed); not lordotic (upper ribs appear to curve forwards and downwards); head turned to the right. X-ray field too large – even right ankle included!

Clinical equipment

Three ECG electrodes, a skin temperature probe, an endotracheal tube (ETT), a nasogastric tube (NGT).

Radiological interpretation

Mediastinum and heart normal. ETT tip at T4. Lung fields cannot be assessed. NGT tip in stomach. Very large translucency overlying most of abdomen suggestive of pneumoperitoneum. Gas in stomach and small bowel.

Conclusion

Gross pneumoperitoneum in a preterm infant on intensive care. A gravity dependent view is unnecessary.

Suggest ETT withdrawn by 1 cm.

CASE STUDY 86: AP VIEW OF ABDOMEN OF INFANT IN SUPINE POSITION WITH VERTICAL BEAM PROJECTION

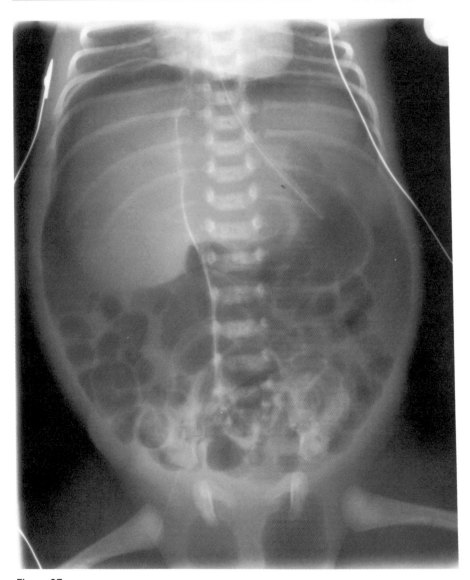

Figure 97

Technical comments

Exposure, positioning and collimation satisfactory.

Clinical equipment

One ECG electrode/lead, nasogastric tube (NGT) and right leg central venous line in situ.

Radiological interpretation

Gross abdominal distension due to a large collection of free gas in peritoneal cavity anteriorly and below diaphragms. Both right and left diaphragms clearly defined/identifiable. Liver on the right. Stomach on the left. NGT tip in stomach. Bowel gas shadows throughout abdomen. Intramural gas – pneumatosis intestinalis – in right lower quadrant. Two large collections of gas in scrotum.

Conclusion

Bowel perforation and massive pneumoperitoneum due to necrotizing enterocolitis in a preterm infant. A gravity dependent view is unnecessary.

CASE STUDY 87: AP VIEW OF ABDOMEN OF PRETERM INFANT IN SUPINE POSITION WITH VERTICAL BEAM PROJECTION

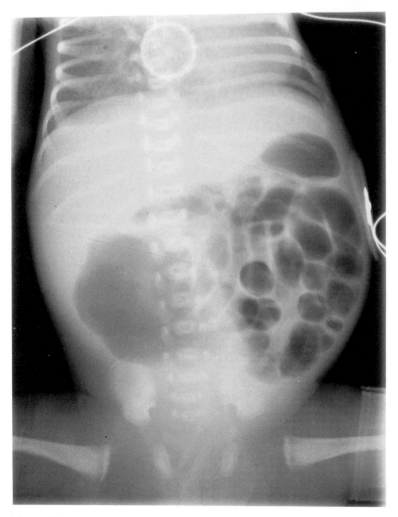

Figure 98a

Technical comments

Exposure satisfactory. Figure 98a markedly rotated to the left. Figure 98b multiple white line artefacts over left abdomen (mattress, sheet, etc.). Infant should have been laid on rectangular foam pad.

AP VIEW OF ABDOMEN OF PRETERM INFANT IN LEFT LATERAL DECUBITUS POSITION WITH HORIZONTAL BEAM PROJECTION

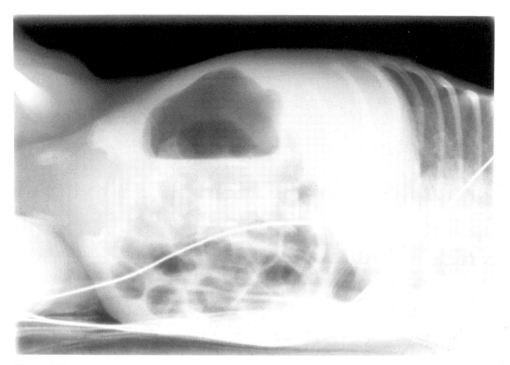

Figure 98b

Clinical equipment

Transcutaneous blood gas monitor probe/sensor base, ECG electrodes/leads and nasogastric tube (NGT) in situ.

Radiological interpretation

Diaphragms intact. Liver on the right. Stomach on the left. NGT tip in stomach. Figure 98a: large gas shadow under liver and displacing bowel gas shadows to the left with no gas in rectum. Figure 98b: large collection of free gas in peritoneal cavity with a large gas fluid level.

Conclusion

Large right abdominal abscess due to bowel perforation in a preterm infant.

CASE STUDY 88: AP VIEW OF ABDOMEN OF INFANT IN SUPINE POSITION WITH VERTICAL BEAM PROJECTION

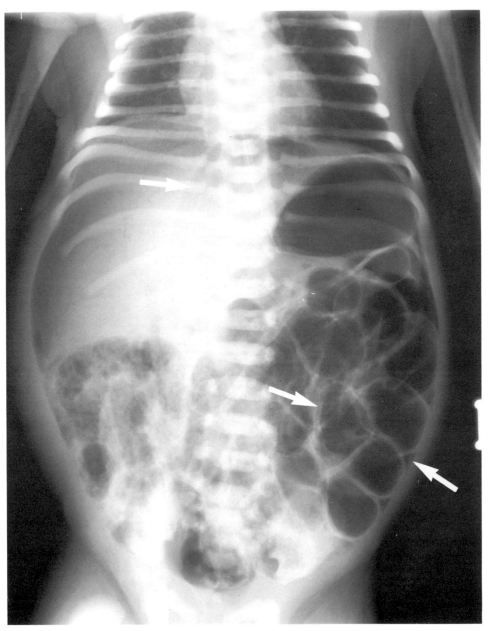

Figure 99

Technical comments

Exposure and positioning satisfactory; lateral collimation good, but too much chest is included.

Clinical equipment

Nasogastric tube (NGT) in situ.

Radiological interpretation

Abdomen grossly distended due to a large collection of free gas in peritoneal cavity outlining falciform ligament (arrows). Diaphragm clearly seen. Liver on the right. Stomach on the left. NGT tip in stomach. Gas in stomach and loops of bowel in left abdomen. Intramural gas – pneumatosis intestinalis (arrow). Gas in portal vein clearly seen against opacity of liver. Free gas in peritoneum between loops of bowel and abdominal wall form pathognomonic translucent triangles (arrow).

Conclusion

Gas in peritoneal cavity and in portal vein: bowel perforation due to necrotizing enterocolitis.

CASE STUDY 89 (A SERIES OF THREE FILMS): AP VIEW OF ABDOMEN OF INFANT IN SUPINE POSITION WITH VERTICAL BEAM PROJECTION

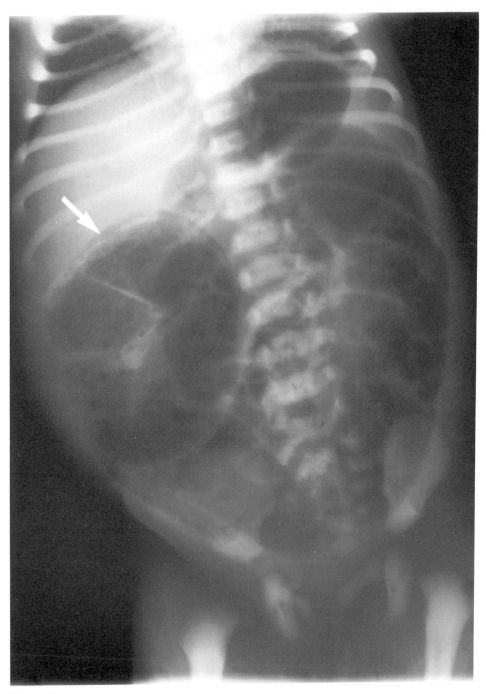

Figure 100a

AP VIEW OF ABDOMEN OF INFANT IN LEFT LATERAL DECUBITUS POSITION WITH HORIZONTAL BEAM PROJECTION

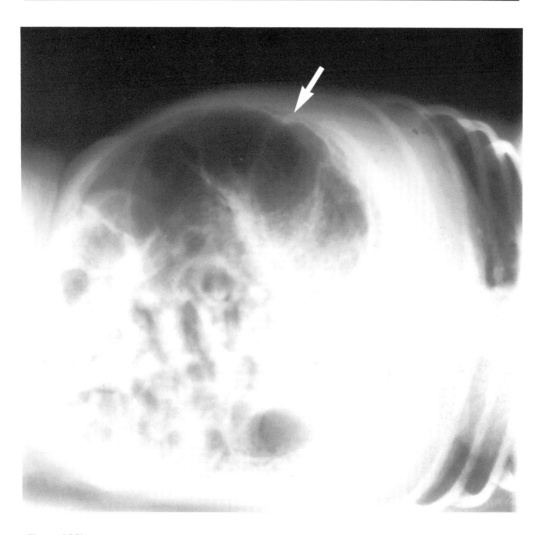

Figure 100b

CASE STUDY 89 (CONTINUED): LATERAL VIEW OF ABDOMEN OF INFANT IN PRONE POSITION WITH HORIZONTAL BEAM PROJECTION

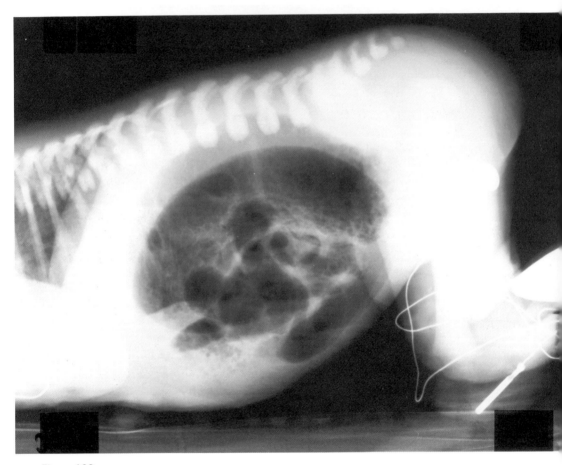

Figure 100c

Technical comments

Exposure satisfactory. Collimation poor in Figure 100c – x-ray field too large; gonad protection is over ankles! 45° foam pad should have been used under hips.

Clinical equipment

Single ECG electrode on upper thigh (Figure 100c).

Radiological interpretation

Figure 100a – Liver on the right. Stomach on the left. Gas throughout bowel with marked gaseous distension of ascending colon, hepatic flexure, splenic flexure and descending colon. Some intramural gas in hepatic flexure (arrow). No gas in rectum.

Figure 100b – Gross gaseous distension of ascending colon and hepatic flexure. Intramural gas present (arrow). No free gas visible in peritoneal cavity.

Figure 100c – Gas in small bowel and gross gaseous distension of colon. Bubbly appearance due to gas–meconium mix.

Conclusion

Necrotizing enterocolitis and sigmoid colon obstruction.
   Differential diagnosis – Hirschsprung's disease, sigmoid atresia, anorectal anomalies.

CASE STUDY 90 (A SERIES OF THREE FILMS): AP VIEW OF ABDOMEN OF TERM INFANT IN SUPINE POSITION WITH VERTICAL BEAM PROJECTION

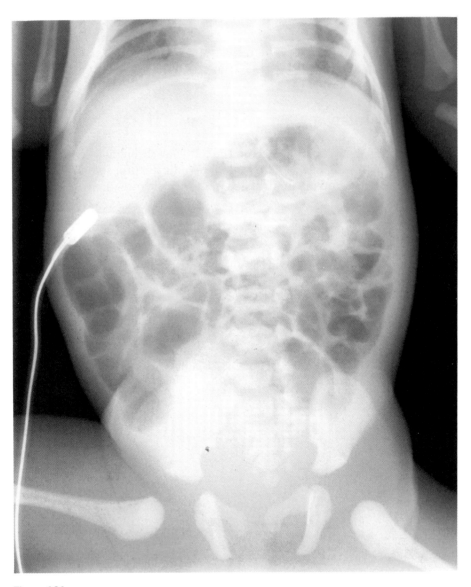

Figure 101a

Technical comments

Figure 101a – Underexposed.

Clinical equipment

Figure 101a – Skin probe/sensor and nasogastric tube (NGT) in situ.

Radiological interpretation

Figure 101a – (5 hours after birth) – diaphragms intact. Liver on the right. Stomach on the left. NGT tip in stomach. Gas throughout small and large bowel. No gas in rectum.

Conclusion

See p. 233.

CASE STUDY 90 (CONTINUED): LATERAL VIEW OF LOWER ABDOMEN AND PELVIS OF TERM INFANT IN INVERTED POSITION WITH HORIZONTAL BEAM PROJECTION

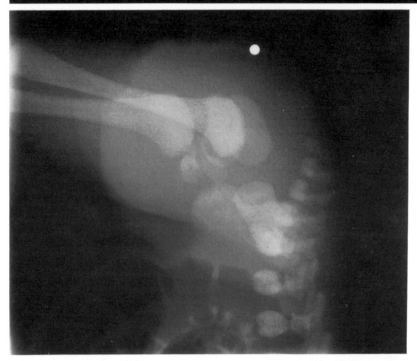

Figure 101b

LATERAL VIEW OF ABDOMEN OF TERM INFANT IN PRONE POSITION WITH HORIZONTAL BEAM PROJECTION

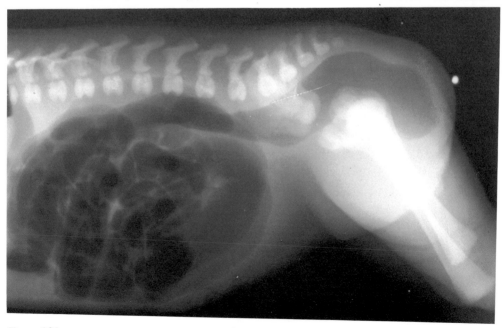

Figure 101c

Technical comments

Figure 101b – Overexposed and rotated (not true lateral of pelvis). Taken too early (5 hours old), must be at least 18 hours old – compare with Figure 101c.

Figure 101c – Satisfactory exposure and positioning. X-ray field too large, upper abdomen included unnecessarily.

Clinical equipment

Figure 101b – Radio-opaque bead on anus.

Figure 101c – Nasogastric tube (NGT) in situ and radio-opaque bead on anus.

Radiological interpretation

Figure 101b – (5 hours after birth) – gas in colon but none in rectum.

Figure 101c – (18 hours after birth) – gross gaseous distension of small and large bowel and rectum.

Conclusion

Infralevator/low imperforate anus.

Note

- Prone horizontal beam projection lateral view (over 45° foam pad (see page 157, Figure 69) has replaced the above inverted view   for this condition.
- Plain films should be delayed until 18–24 hours of age to allow gas to extend into upper rectal pouch.
- High anorectal anomalies may be associated with a rectovesicular, rectourethral or rectovaginal fistula.
- Associated anomalies are common: vertebral (28%), central nervous system (18%), heart (9%) and gastrointestinal tract (9%).

CASE STUDY 91: AP VIEW OF ABDOMEN AND LOWER CHEST OF INFANT IN SUPINE POSITION WITH VERTICAL BEAM PROJECTION

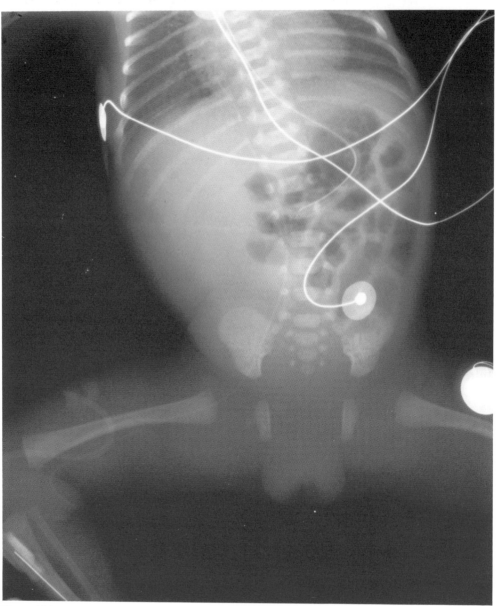

Figure 102

Technical comments

Exposure satisfactory (spine visible through heart shadow). Not rotated (iliac bones symmetrical). ECG leads should have been removed from field of interest. No need to x-ray leg for insertion site. Gonads irradiated.

Clinical equipment

Three ECG electrodes/leads, a skin probe/sensor, a nasogastric tube (NGT) and a central venous line (CVL) in situ.

Radiological interpretation

Diaphragms intact. Liver on the right. NGT tip in stomach on the left. No bowel gas in right abdomen. Bowel gas shadows in left abdomen appear normal. No signs of intramural gas. No gas in rectum. Right leg CVL passing up inferior vena cava into heart.

Conclusion

Space occupying mass in right abdomen of preterm infant.
   Suggest ultrasound examination of right abdomen and kidneys.

CASE STUDY 92: AP VIEW OF ABDOMEN, INCLUDING CHEST, OF INFANT IN SUPINE POSITION WITH VERTICAL BEAM PROJECTION

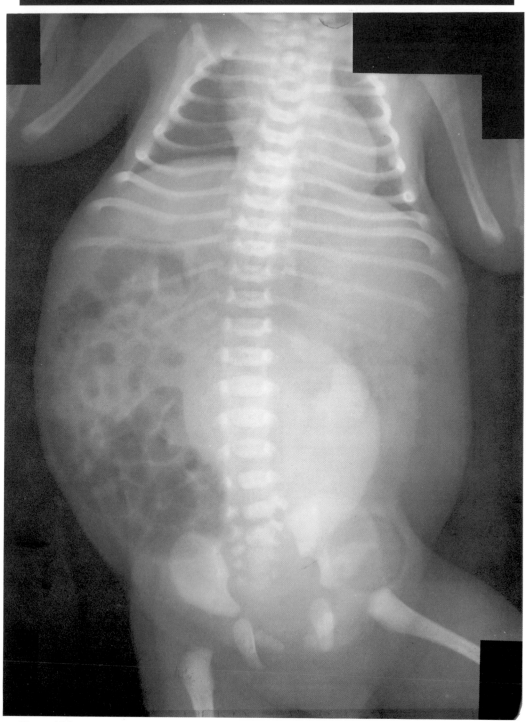

Figure 103

Technical comments

Exposure unsatisfactory (grey film, no contrast or detail); expiratory film (5 posterior rib ends visible above right diaphragm); not markedly rotated (rib cage symmetrical appearance); grossly lordotic (upper ribs appear to curve forwards and upwards) because centring is on abdomen. The chest has been irradiated unnecessarily; this distorted view is not diagnostic.

Clinical equipment

Nil.

Radiological interpretation

Heart and mediastinum appear normal. Small lung fields which appear clear. Massive abdominal distension. Diaphragms intact. Liver on the right. Stomach position indeterminate. Normal intestinal gas shadows displaced to the right abdomen by large mass which occupies whole of left and central abdomen and which is more radio-opaque in central abdomen. Note artefact over right hip caused by incubator hole.

Conclusion

Probable large urachal cyst and hydronephrosis in an infant with prune-belly syndrome (hypotonic, hypoplastic anterior abdominal wall musculature, undescended testes and urinary tract anomalies, especially urethral obstruction).

Clinical Equipment and Artefacts

Neonatal intensive care requires much high technology equipment and techniques with access to body surfaces, arteries, veins, trachea, gastrointestinal/urinary tracts and body cavities. This equipment may be the cause of iatrogenic disease or trauma, especially if incorrectly positioned. **A post-insertion radiograph to check positioning of catheters/lines/tubes is essential and must be viewed at once. A film showing a dangerously misplaced tube (e.g. endotracheal tube in right main bronchus, Figures 31a, 32a and 35, or in oesophagus, Figures 55 and 121) must not be left on the ward to await a doctor's return, possibly hours later. It is the responsibility of the radiographer and/or nurse in charge to contact the doctor urgently, even if the doctor is busy on another ward. Prompt action is life saving.**

After positioning the infant and before exposing the film the radiographer, with the nurse's help and advice, should check that:

1. Movable equipment (e.g. ECG leads, ventilator tubing) is cleared from the x-ray field.

2. No misleading shadows, e.g. incubator hole (Figure 124), apnoea mattress, etc., appear on the film.

A radiograph taken to localize an umbilical arterial catheter (UAC) must include the whole abdomen and chest. (Chest/upper abdomen or abdomen alone are often mistakenly requested, see Figure 112.)

- The recommended position of the UAC tip is either low (L3–4) or high (T6–10).

- The chest must be seen in case the catheter tip is sited far too high (Figures 112 and 113).

- The U-bend of the UAC's course (Figures 110, 111, 112 and 113) must be visualized in the lower abdomen to check it is not in the umbilical vein by mistake. Arterial and venous catheters are most clearly differentiated on a lateral view of the abdomen. From the umbilicus, arterial catheters pass down into the pelvis before returning along the posterior abdominal wall (Figure 115), whereas venous catheters pass directly up the ductus venosus to the inferior vena cava.

CASE STUDY 93: AP VIEW OF PRETERM CHEST AND UPPER ABDOMEN

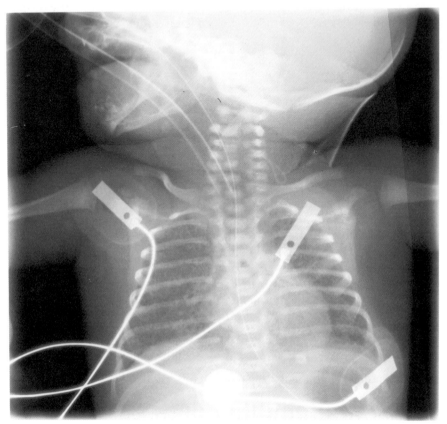

Figure 104

Technical comments

Exposure satisfactory (spine visible through heart shadow); partial inspiratory film but acceptable (8 posterior rib ends visible above right diaphragm); no significant rotation (anterior rib ends symmetrically placed); mildly lordotic (upper ribs horizontal); head facing to the right. The ECG leads should have been cleared from the field of interest.

Clinical equipment

A transcutaneous oxygen sensor, endotracheal tube (ETT), nasogastric tube (NGT), left scalp central venous line (CVL) and three ECG electrodes in situ. Note strapping on neck. The ECG pads are apparent at the very low exposures required for premature infants and therefore should be placed on the shoulders and abdomen clear of the lung fields.

Radiological interpretation

Mediastinum and heart appear normal. ETT tip at T1. Lung fields show some reticulation and opacification, probably due to poor aeration. Left scalp CVL curled/doubled back on itself at the junction of jugular and subclavian veins. NGT passing into stomach but location of tip off the film. No gas under diaphragms. Gastric air bubble present. Left paravertebral small round opacity.

Conclusion

Normal heart and lungs in a very preterm infant on intensive care. Calcification probably left adrenal gland.
   Recommend adjustment of central venous line.

Note

▪ The ECG pads are semiopaque and their edges should not be mistaken for lung markings or a pneumothorax 'edge'.

CASE STUDY 94: AP VIEW OF CHEST AND UPPER ABDOMEN OF A PRETERM INFANT

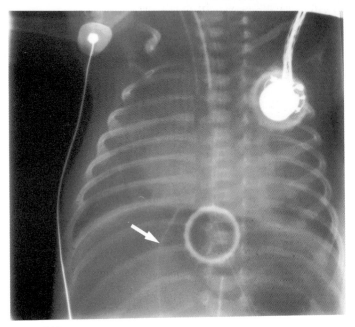

Figure 105

Technical comments

Overexposed (dark film and no lung detail visible); partial inspiratory film (8 posterior rib ends visible above right diaphragm); markedly rotated to the right (rib cage asymmetrical with apparently longer ribs on the right and asymmetrically placed anterior rib ends); not lordotic (upper ribs appear to curve forwards and downwards); head facing right.

Clinical equipment

One ECG electrode, a transcutaneous blood gas monitor probe/sensor base and another with probe/sensor in place, endotracheal tube (ETT), umbilical catheter and nasogastric tube (NGT) in situ. The probe/sensor should not have been placed over the left lung apex.

Radiological interpretation

Mediastinum, heart and trachea rotated to the right. ETT tip at T3. No lung field detail visible on this overexposed film. NGT passing into abdomen but tip off the film. Hypertranslucency of upper abdomen with ligamentum teres clearly outlined (arrow).

Conclusion

Technically inadequate film with lung apex obscured by skin probe/sensor. Upper abdominal appearance suggestive of gross pneumoperitoneum.
  Suggest:

1. Repeat chest x-ray with above skin probe/sensor removed and correct exposure and positioning.

2. Lateral view of abdomen in dorsal decubitus position with a horizontal beam projection to confirm pneumoperitoneum.

CASE STUDY 95: AP VIEW OF CHEST AND UPPER ABDOMEN OF INFANT

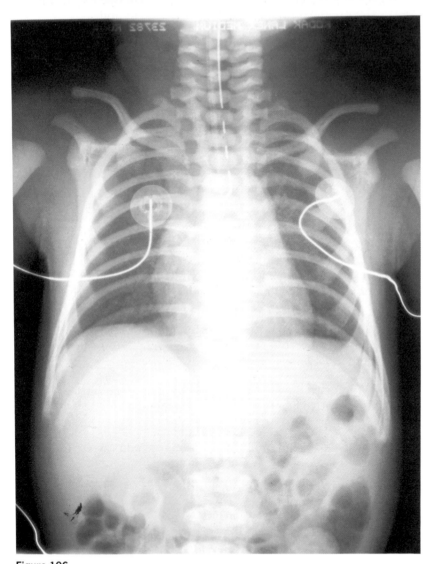

Figure 106

Technical comments

Exposure satisfactory (spine visible through heart shadow); inspiratory film (9 posterior rib ends visible above right diaphragm); not rotated (anterior rib ends symmetrically placed); not lordotic (upper ribs appear to curve forwards and downwards).

Clinical equipment

Two ECG electrodes and a 'nasogastric tube' in situ. The electrodes should have been moved to shoulders away from field of interest.

Radiological interpretation

Mediastinum, heart, lungs and abdomen appear normal. No vertebral abnormalities. Cervical ribs present. Only 11 ribs present on both sides. NGT tip in mid-oesophagus. Black artefact (which is photographic) over right abdomen.

Conclusion

High NGT tip either due to incomplete insertion of NGT or to oesphageal atresia with a fistulous connection between the tracheobronchial tree and the lower oesophageal pouch.

Note

■ Rib abnormalities.

Suggest:

1. Re-insertion of NGT (French gauge 12).
2. Repeat chest x-ray, to check NGT position.

CASE STUDY 96: AP VIEW OF CHEST AND UPPER ABDOMEN OF PRETERM INFANT

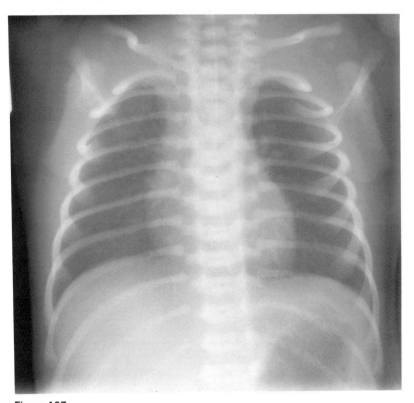

Figure 107

Technical comments

Exposure unsatisfactory (grey film with little contrast); partial inspiratory film (8 posterior rib ends visible above right diaphragm); rotated to the right (anterior rib ends asymmetrically placed); lordotic (upper ribs appear to curve forwards and upwards).

Clinical equipment

Nasogastric tube in situ.

Radiological interpretation

Mediastinum, heart and lung fields appear normal. Diaphragms, liver and air in stomach appear normal. NGT tip in lower oesophagus at T8.

Conclusion

NGT tip placed high in lower oesophagus of preterm infant.

Suggest NGT is inserted further and if no acidic gastric aspirate obtained, the radiograph should be repeated.

Note

■ Neonatal radiographs must be examined carefully for positioning of clinical equipment which may not be obvious.

CASE STUDY 97: AP VIEW OF CHEST AND ABDOMEN OF PRETERM INFANT

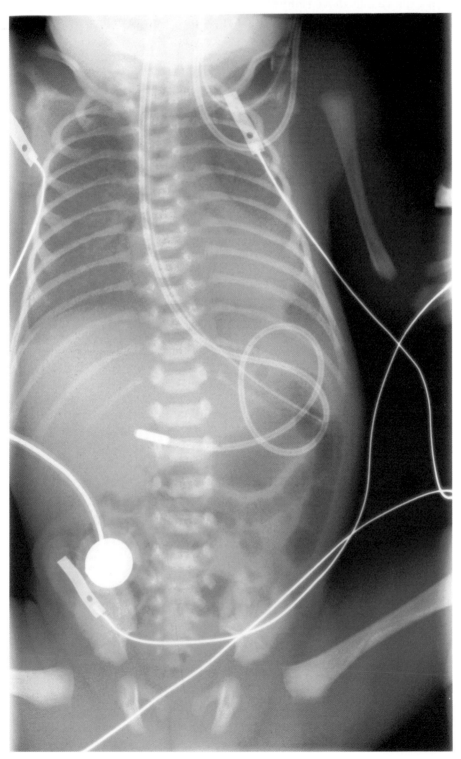

Figure 108

Technical comments

Exposure satisfactory (spine visible through heart shadow); inspiratory film (9
posterior rib ends visible above right diaphragm); not rotated (anterior rib ends
symmetrically placed); not lordotic (upper ribs appear to curve forwards and
downwards); head facing forwards. Lateral collimation of x-ray beam inaccurate.
Enteral tubes should have been removed from overlying left lung apex.

Clinical equipment

Two ECG electrodes, a skin probe, a nasogastric tube (NGT) and a nasojejunal
tube (NJT) in situ. ECG electrodes should have been removed from overlying left
lung apex. Other electrodes/skin probes obscure the right lower abdomen and
should be moved to sides of abdomen or upper thighs away from field of interest.

Radiological interpretation

Mediastinum and heart normal. Air in trachea and main bronchi clearly seen.
Good lung detail – appears normal. Left lung apex obscured by overlying clinical
equipment. NGT tip in stomach. NJT metal tip at pylorus. Diaphragms visible.
Liver on the right. Stomach on the left. Normal small and large bowel gas shadows
but **overlying clinical equipment obscuring right lower abdomen – area
where necrotizing enterocolitis is common – should have been resited**. Air
in rectum.

Conclusion

NGT and NJT appropriately sited for enteral feeding in preterm infant.
   If abdominal distension develops suggest AP view of abdomen in supine position
with vertical beam projection to exclude early radiological signs of necrotizing
enterocolitis.

CASE STUDY 98: AP VIEW OF CHEST AND ABDOMEN OF PRETERM INFANT

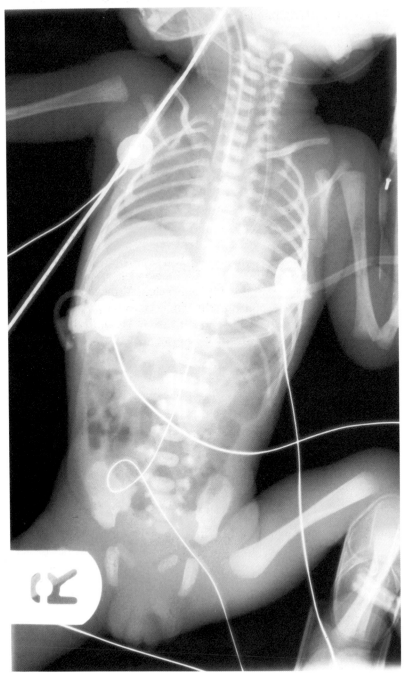

Figure 109

Technical comments

Exposure satisfactory (spine visible through heart shadow); expiratory film (7 posterior rib ends visible above right diaphragm); rotated to the right (anterior rib ends asymmetrically placed and asymmetry of rib cage with right ribs appearing longer); not lordotic (upper ribs appear to curve downwards and forwards); head facing to the right. Poor collimation with limbs unnecessarily irradiated. Monitor leads and nasogastric tube (NGT) female connectors should have been moved from field of interest.

Clinical equipment

Three ECG electrodes, endotracheal tube (ETT), NGT and umbilical catheter (UC) electrode in situ. The ECG electrodes should be placed on shoulders and thighs away from field of interest.

Radiological interpretation

Mediastinum, heart and trachea rotated to right. ETT tip at T4. Inadequate film for comment on lung fields. UC electrode tip at T10. No clear U-bend to prove it is in the artery. Right diaphragm visible. Left diaphragm obscured by electrode and NGT connector. Liver on the right. Stomach on the left. NGT tip in first part of duodenum. Normal bowel gas shadows. No gas in rectum.

Conclusion

Technically inadequate film for assessment of infant. Site of UC equivocal.
   Suggest:

1 Withdraw ETT by 1 cm.

2. Withdraw NGT by 2 cm.

3. Reposition electrodes.

4. Repeat chest and abdomen film with faults itemized above corrected.

5. Lateral abdomen to locate site of UC (see Figure 115).

CASE STUDY 99: AP VIEW OF CHEST AND ABDOMEN OF A PRETERM INFANT

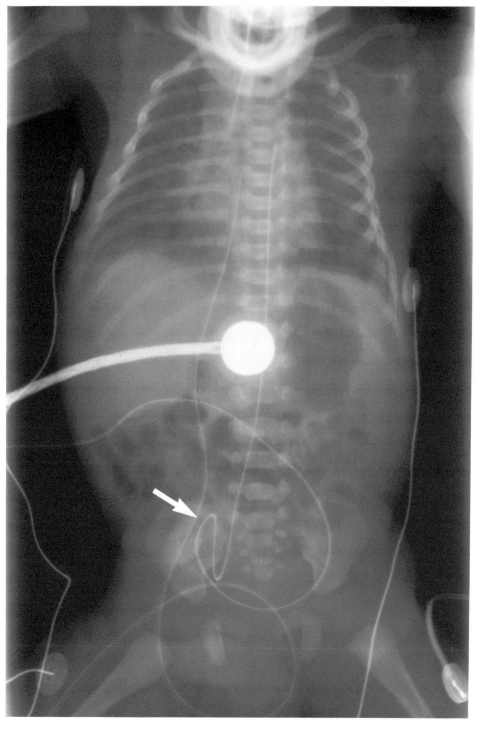

Figure 110

Technical comments

Overexposed (dark film with no lung detail); inspiratory film (9 posterior rib ends visible above right diaphragm); rotated to the right (rib cage asymmetrical with apparently longer ribs on the right and asymmetrically placed anterior rib ends); not lordotic (anterior rib ends appear to curve forwards and downwards); head facing forwards. Loops of umbilical catheters should have been removed from rectal/scrotal area. Poor collimation: gonads irradiated unnecessarily.

Clinical equipment

Three ECG electrodes, a skin probe/sensor, a transcutaneous blood gas monitor skin probe/sensor, endotracheal tube (ETT), umbilical venous catheter (UVC) and umbilical arterial catheter (UAC) in situ. Blood gas monitor skin probe/sensor should not have been placed over midline where it could have obscured catheter tip position.

Radiological interpretation

Mediastinum, heart and trachea rotated to the right. ETT tip at T5 – bifurcation of trachea. Lung field detail cannot be seen on this overexposed film. UVC tip at T7 and UAC tip at T5–6. Note location of umbilicus (arrow) and U-bend of UAC in contradistinction to straight course of UVC. Diaphragms visible. Liver on the right. Stomach on the left. Bowel gas shadows appear normal. No gas in rectum.

Conclusion

Technically unsatisfactory chest x-ray – overexposed and rotated. ETT tip too low. High UVC and UAC in a preterm infant on intensive care.
Suggest:

1. Withdraw ETT by 1 cm.

2. Withdraw UVC by 2 cm.

3. Withdraw UAC by 2.5 cm.

4. Resite transcutaneous probe/sensor.

5. Repeat x-ray of chest and abdomen with correct exposure and positioning.

CASE STUDY 100: AP VIEW OF CHEST AND ABDOMEN OF MARKEDLY PRETERM INFANT

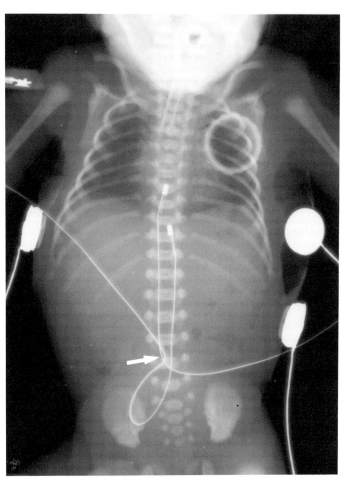

Figure 111

Technical comments

Exposure unsatisfactory for chest (no lung detail), satisfactory for abdomen; part inspiratory film (8 posterior rib ends visible above right diaphragm); not rotated (anterior rib ends symmetrically placed); not lordotic (upper ribs appear to curve forwards and downwards); head facing forwards.

Clinical equipment

Four skin probe/sensors, one transcutaneous blood gas monitor probe/sensor base, umbilical venous catheter (UVC) electrode and umbilical arterial catheter (UAC) electrode in situ. The probe/sensor base should be resited to right upper or lateral abdomen away from field of interest.

Radiological interpretation

Mediastinum, heart and lungs appear normal. ETT tip at T4 – bifurcation of trachea. Note position of catheter entry at umbilicus (arrow). UVC passes directly upwards into inferior vena cava whereas UAC passes through a downward pelvic loop before ascending the abdominal and thoracic aorta. UVC electrode tip at T7. UAC electrode tip at T9. Only a few bowel gas shadows in abdomen.

Conclusion

Correctly placed UVC electrode and UAC electrode in a markedly preterm infant on intensive care. ETT tip too low.

Suggest ETT withdrawal by 0.5 cm.

CASE STUDY 101: AP VIEW OF ABDOMEN OF PRETERM INFANT IN SUPINE POSITION WITH VERTICAL BEAM PROJECTION

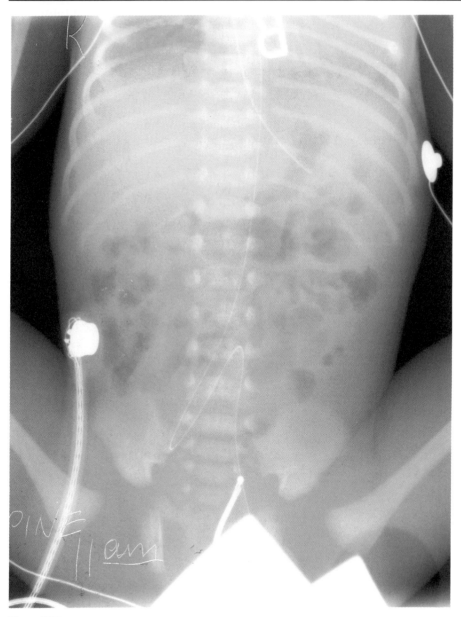

Figure 112

Technical comments

Underexposed film (too pale); incorrectly placed gonad protection and letter R.

Clinical equipment

Two ECG electrodes, three ECG leads, skin probe/sensor, nasogastric tube (NGT), rectal probe, umbilical arterial catheter (UAC) and gonad shield in situ.

Radiological interpretation

Liver on the right. NGT passing into stomach on the left. Bowel gas pattern poorly shown on this underexposed film. No gas in rectum which is partly obscured by gonad shield. UAC passing through characteristic U-bend in lower abdomen into abdominal and thoracic aorta with position of tip not shown. Incubator hole translucency over upper left thigh.

Conclusion

Technically unsatisfactory film of abdomen and for localization of position of tip of UAC.
  Suggest chest x-ray to locate tip of UAC.

Note:

- Post-UAC insertion films to check positioning should include whole abdomen (to ensure presence of U-bend) and whole chest (to locate tip).
- Gonad protection can obscure rectum.

CASE STUDY 102: AP VIEW OF PRETERM CHEST AND ABDOMEN

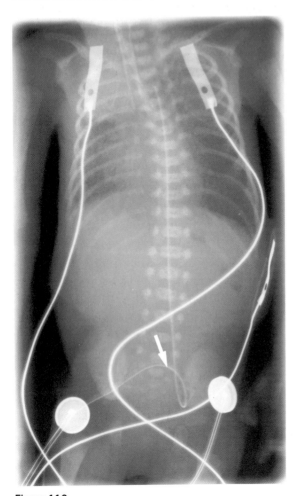

Figure 113

Technical comments

Exposure satisfactory (spine visible through heart shadow); inspiratory film (9 posterior rib ends visible above the right diaphragm); significantly rotated to the right (rib cage appears asymmetrical and anterior rib ends are asymmetrically placed); not lordotic (upper ribs appear to curve forwards and downwards); ECG leads should have been cleared from field of interest.

Clinical equipment

Resuscitation (shouldered Coles) endotracheal tube (ETT), umbilical arterial catheter (UAC), three ECG electrodes and two skin probes in situ. ECG electrodes overlying lung apices should have been placed on shoulders and abdomen clear of lung fields.

Radiological interpretation

Mediastinum and heart shadow appear displaced to the right by the rotation. ETT tip at T4, i.e. at the tracheal bifurcation. Right upper lobe collapse consolidation. Otherwise lung fields appear normal. UAC enters umbilicus (arrow), passes down into pelvis before ascending aorta with tip at T3. Abdomen shows few gas shadows.

Conclusion

Right upper lobe collapse consolidation in a very preterm infant on intensive care. Recommend withdrawal of ETT by 1 cm and UAC by 2.5 cm.

Note

▪ The ECG pads are semiopaque at the very low exposures required for premature infants, and they should not be mistaken for lung markings or the 'edge' of a pneumothorax.

CASE STUDY 103: AP VIEW OF CHEST AND UPPER ABDOMEN OF PRETERM INFANT

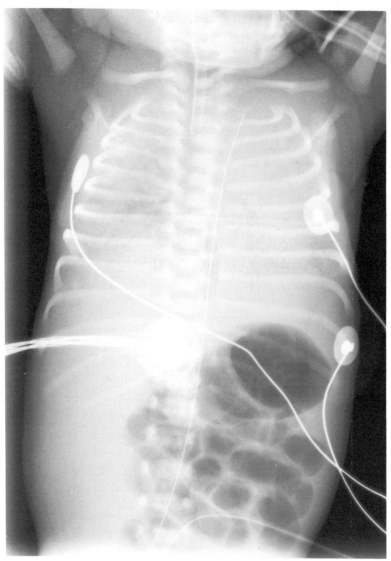

Figure 114

Technical comments

Exposure satisfactory (spine visible through heart shadow); lungs not inflated; rotated to the left (asymmetry of rib cage with longer ribs on the left); grossly lordotic (upper 6 ribs appear to curve forwards and upwards); head facing forwards. Monitor lead should have been cleared from field of interest. Infant's arms should not be held up beside head (causes lordotic projection).

Clinical equipment

Three ECG leads, a transcutaneous blood gas monitor probe/sensor, Coles shouldered resuscitation/endotracheal tube (ETT) and umbilical arterial catheter (UAC) in situ.

Radiological interpretation

ETT tip at T1. Homogeneous opacification (white out) of chest with minimal aeration of mid right lung field. UAC tip at T1. Position of diaphragms not identifiable. Liver on the right. Stomach on the left. Normal bowel gas shadows only in left abdomen. Right abdomen opaque.

Conclusion

Technically poor film: rotated and markedly lordotic. High UAC in a preterm infant who is on intensive care and who has markedly inadequate ventilation.
   Suggest:

1. Adjust ventilation.

2. Withdraw UAC by 5 cm.

3. Repeat chest x-ray correctly positioned.

4. Once cardiorespiratory status is stabilized, AP views of abdomen supine with vertical beam projection and left lateral decubitus (right side up) position with horizontal beam projection to define right abdominal opacity.

CASE STUDY 104: LATERAL VIEW OF ABDOMEN OF PRETERM INFANT IN DORSAL DECUBITUS POSITION WITH HORIZONTAL BEAM PROJECTION

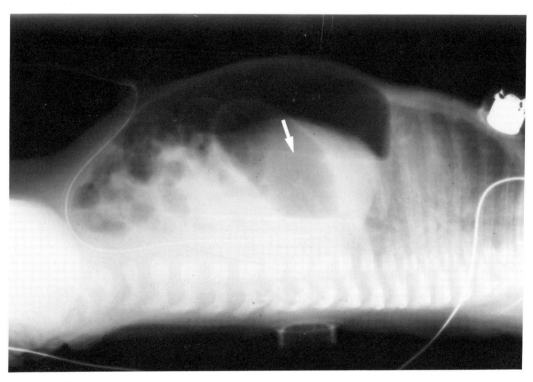

Figure 115

Technical comments

Exposure satisfactory. (*Note:* anterior abdominal wall requires less exposure than posterior abdomen.) Some rotation – anterior rib ends do not coincide.

Clinical equipment

A transcutaneous blood gas monitor probe/sensor and a separate base, ECG lead and an umbilical arterial catheter (UAC) in situ.

Radiological interpretation

Abdominal distension caused by large collection of free gas in peritoneal cavity. Ligamentum teres clearly outlined (arrow). Gaseous distension of stomach. Note characteristic course of UAC.

Conclusion

Gross pneumoperitoneum in a preterm infant with a UAC in situ.

CASE STUDY 105: AP VIEW OF CHEST OF PRETERM INFANT

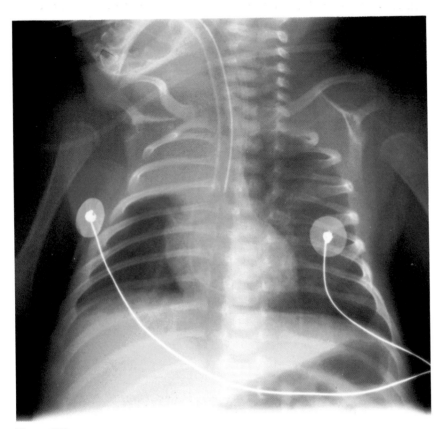

Figure 116

Technical comments

Exposure satisfactory (spine visible through heart shadow); partial inspiratory film (8 ribs visible above right diaphragm); marked rotation to the right (asymmetry of rib cage with longer ribs on the right); slightly lordotic (upper ribs almost horizontal); head turned to the right which invariably causes rotation. Tubing seen across neck should have been cleared.

Clinical equipment

Two ECG electrodes, endotracheal tube (ETT), nasogastric tube (NGT) and central venous line (CVL) in situ. The left chest electrode should have been placed away from the field of interest, e.g. on left shoulder.

Radiological interpretation

Mediastinum and heart rotated to the right. ETT tip at T4 – at tracheal bifurcation. Right upper lobe collapse consolidation with increased translucency of right lower lung field. Left lung field clear. Left arm CVL tip in right ventricle. NGT tip in lower oesophagus. Liver on the right. Stomach on the left.

Conclusion

Right upper lobe collapse consolidation in a preterm infant on intensive care. Suggest:

1. Withdraw ETT by 1 cm.

2. Withdraw CVL by 2.5 cm.

3. Insert NGT further so that tip is in stomach.

CASE STUDY 106: AP VIEW OF PRETERM CHEST

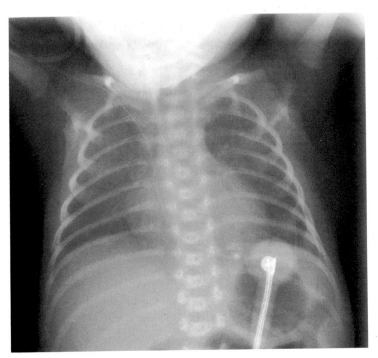

Figure 117

Technical comments

Exposure satisfactory (spine visible through heart shadow and lung detail present); part inspiratory film (8 posterior rib ends visible above right diaphragm); not rotated (anterior rib ends symmetrically placed); not lordotic (upper ribs appear to curve forwards and downwards); head facing forwards.

Clinical equipment

A transcutaneous blood gas monitor probe/sensor, a nasogastric tube (NGT) and a central venous line (CVL) in situ.

Radiological interpretation

Mediastinum, heart, lungs and upper abdomen all appear normal. NGT tip in stomach. CVL tip position defined by contrast injection.

Conclusion

CVL tip in right ventricle of preterm infant.

Note

■ Contrast medium should be used only with radiologist's approval.

CASE STUDY 107: AP VIEW OF CHEST AND UPPER ABDOMEN OF A MARKEDLY PRETERM INFANT

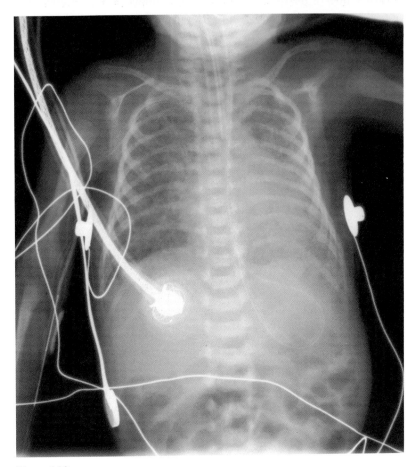

Figure 118

Technical comments

Exposure satisfactory (spine visible through heart shadow); inspiratory film (9 posterior rib ends visible above the right diaphragm); not significantly rotated (anterior rib ends symmetrically placed); not lordotic (upper ribs appear to curve forwards and downwards); head facing forwards. Lateral collimation inaccurate: no need to x-ray arm for insertion site. Monitor leads should have been cleared from field of interest.

Clinical equipment

Two ECG electrodes, a transcutaneous blood gas monitor probe/sensor, another skin probe/sensor, endotracheal tube (ETT), nasogastric tube (NGT) and central venous line (CVL) in situ.

Radiological interpretation

Mediastinum and heart poorly visualized. ETT tip at T5. Patchy consolidation of both lung fields. CVL tip in right internal jugular vein. Right diaphragm visible; left diaphragm poorly seen. Liver on the right. NGT tip has doubled up in stomach on the left so that tip has re-entered lower oesophagus. Bowel gas shadows appear normal.

Conclusion

Incorrectly placed ETT, NGT and CVL in a markedly preterm infant on intensive care with lung field appearances compatible with either infection or early bronchopulmonary dysplasia.
　　Suggest:

1. Withdraw ETT by 1 cm.

2. Withdraw NGT by 2.5 cm.

3. Withdraw CVL by 2.5 cm.

CASE STUDY 108: PA VIEW OF CHEST AND UPPER ABDOMEN OF INFANT

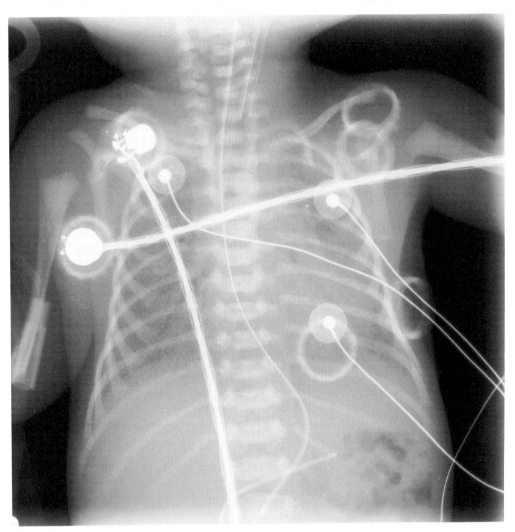

Figure 119

Technical comments

Exposure satisfactory (spine visible through heart shadow); inspiratory film (9 posterior rib ends visible above right diaphragm); rotated to the left (anterior rib ends asymmetrically placed); not lordotic (upper ribs appear to curve forwards and downwards); head facing left. Monitor leads should have been removed from field of interest, if possible. *Note:* this film was taken with infant prone, so rotation is unavoidable and leads are probably underneath infant.

Clinical equipment

Three ECG electrodes, four transcutaneous blood gas monitor probe/sensor bases and two probe/sensors, endotracheal tube (ETT) and nasogastric tube (NGT) in situ. The three ECG leads should have been placed on the shoulders and a thigh.

Radiological interpretation

Mediastinum, heart and trachea rotated to the left. ETT tip at T1. Air in trachea and main bronchi clearly seen. Homogeneous opacification of both visible lung fields. Diaphragm unclearly seen. Liver on the right. NGT tip in stomach on the left.

Conclusion

Lung field appearances compatible with respiratory distress caused by either hyaline membrane disease or group B streptococcal infection in an infant on intensive care. The view is unnecessarily cluttered by clinical equipment.

Suggest repeat chest x-ray with relocation of clinical equipment and with correct positioning.

CASE STUDY 109: AP VIEW OF CHEST AND ABDOMEN OF A MARKEDLY PRETERM INFANT

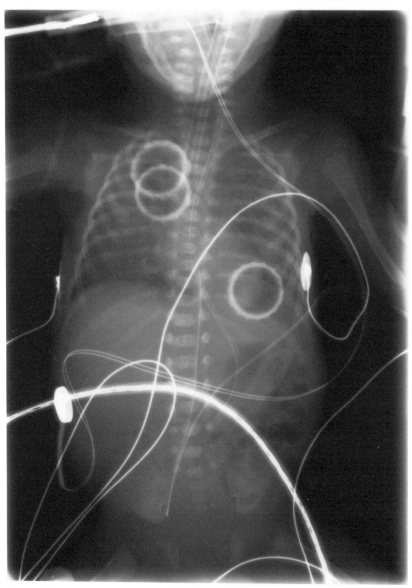

Figure 120

Technical comments

Overexposed film for lung detail; overinflated (10 posterior rib ends visible above right diaphragm); not significantly rotated (anterior rib ends symmetrically placed); not lordotic (upper ribs appear to curve forwards and downwards); head facing forwards. Multiple monitor leads should have been cleared from the field of interest.

Clinical equipment

Two ECG electrodes, a skin probe/sensor, three transcutaneous blood gas monitor probe/sensor bases, endotracheal tube (ETT), nasogastric tube (NGT), umbilical arterial catheter (UAC) and a right arm central venous line (CVL) in situ. Multiple sensor bases should have been placed away from the field of interest.

Radiological interpretation

This exceptionally poor film is of no value in assessing this infant's condition.
    ETT tip at T3–4. NGT tip in stomach. UAC tip at T9. Position of CVL tip unclear.

Conclusion

Technically overexposed film of preterm chest and abdomen which is cluttered (unnecessarily) with clinical equipment, obscuring radiological information.
    Suggest appropriate relocation of clinical equipment and repeat film with correct exposure.

CASE STUDY 110: AP VIEW OF PRETERM CHEST AND UPPER ABDOMEN

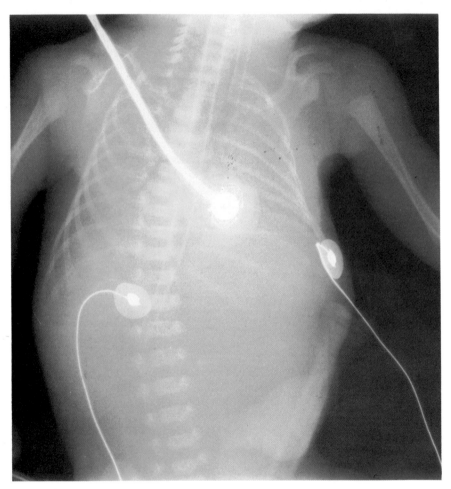

Figure 121

Technical comments

Exposure unsatisfactory (grey film, no contrast or detail); inspiratory film (9 posterior rib ends visible above right diaphragm); marked rotation to the left (anterior rib ends asymmetrically placed and posterior ribs appear longer on the left); not lordotic (upper ribs appear to curve forwards and downwards); arms irradiated unnecessarily.

Clinical equipment

Two ECG electrodes, a transcutaneous blood gas monitor skin probe/sensor and Coles endotracheal tubes (ETT) in situ.

Radiological interpretation

Technically unacceptable film. ETT tip in trachea at T3. Another ETT appears to be in oesophagus with tip in stomach.

Conclusion

ETT obviously misplaced in oesophagus. *Note:* not so obvious in a non-rotated film as endotracheal tubes would be partly superimposed.
   Suggest:

1. Need to check ETT not lying under infant.

2. Repeat chest x-ray with correct exposure and positioning.

3. Removal of misplaced ETT.

Note

No record of misplaced ETT during resuscitation. Infant transferred with both Coles ETTs in situ. Misplaced ETT not discovered for 3 days (weekend) at receiving hospital.

CASE STUDY 111: AP VIEW OF PRETERM CHEST AND UPPER ABDOMEN

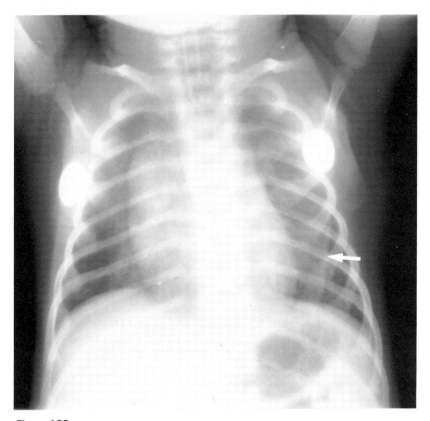

Figure 122

Technical comment

Exposure satisfactory (spine visible through heart shadow); part inspiration (8/9 posterior rib ends visible above right diaphragm); rotation to the right (anterior rib ends asymmetrically placed and posterior ribs appear longer on the right); not lordotic (upper ribs appear to curve forwards and downwards).

Clinical equipment

Two ECG electrodes and endotracheal tube (ETT) in situ.

Radiological interpretation

Mediastinum and heart rotated to the right. ETT tip at T1–2. Curvilinear line in left lower lung field (arrow) with increased translucency and no lung markings seen external to it. Translucency of right and left lung fields approximately equal. No other abnormalities of lung fields. Liver on the right. Stomach on the left.

Conclusion

Skin crease or small left pneumothorax in a preterm infant on ventilation.

Suggest AP view of chest in right lateral decubitus position (left side up) with a horizontal beam projection (see Figure 30c and d) to exclude a small pneumothorax.

Note

■ Symmetry of position of ends of clavicles is **not** a good index of rotation.

CASE STUDY 112: AP VIEW OF PRETERM CHEST AND UPPER ABDOMEN

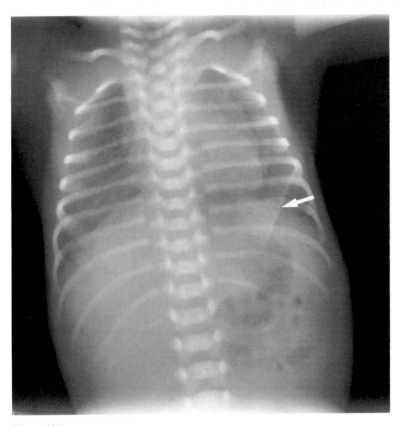

Figure 123

Technical comments

Exposure satisfactory (spine clearly visible through heart shadow); expiratory film (7 posterior rib ends visible on the right); not rotated (anterior rib ends symmetrically placed); lordotic (upper rib ends turned up); head position off the film.

Clinical equipment

Nil.

Radiological interpretation

Mediastinum and heart not displaced. Left lower lung field diagonal straight line (arrow) crossing diaphragm. Skin crease suggested if lung markings can be seen distally/externally: this artefact can sometimes mimic a pneumothorax. Lung fields appear normal. Diaphragms, liver, stomach and bowel gas shadows appear normal.

Conclusion

Left lower lung field skin crease in an otherwise apparently normal chest and upper abdomen of a preterm infant.
   Suggest:

1. Repeat film on inspiration.

2. If line present on repeat film, an AP view of chest in right lateral decubitus position (left side up) with a horizontal beam projection (see Figure 30c and d) will exclude a small pneumothorax.

CASE STUDY 113: AP VIEW OF PRETERM CHEST AND UPPER ABDOMEN

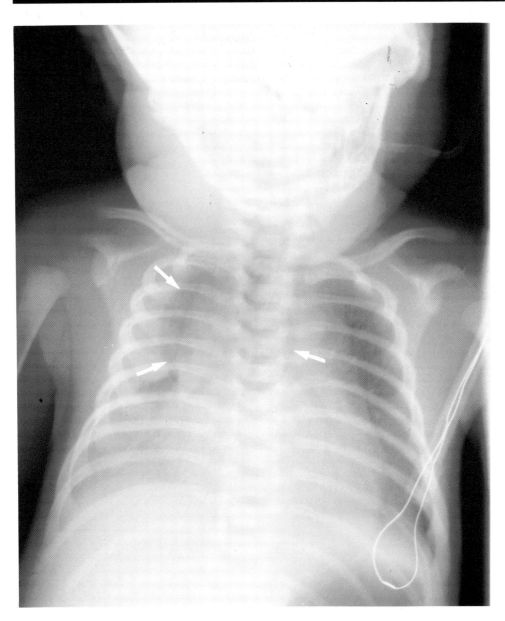

Figure 124

Technical comments

Exposure unsatisfactory (pale film, poor contrast, poor lung detail); inspiratory film (9–10 posterior rib ends visible above right diaphragm); slightly rotated to the left (anterior rib ends asymmetrically placed); not lordotic (upper ribs appear to curve forwards and downwards); head tilted but facing forwards; upper face and eyes irradiated unnecessarily. Lead/wire should have been removed from x-ray field and infant from underneath the incubator hole (see p. 5).

Clinical equipment

Nasal catheter in situ.

Radiological equipment

Wide upper mediastinum probably due to thymus. Heart slightly enlarged (cardiothoracic ratio 0.6). Only upper liver included and therefore not possible to exclude hepatomegaly due to congestive heart failure. Air bronchogram overlying heart shadow. Circular translucency over upper right mediastinum and lung field (arrows). Homogeneous opacification of right lung compared to left lung field. Liver on the right. Stomach on the left. Nasal catheter not seen in oesophagus.

Conclusion

Circular translucency artefact due to incubator hole. **This must NOT be mistaken for an air leak.** The radiograph does not conclusively indicate/identify heart or lung pathology.

Suggest repeat x-ray, with correct exposure, of chest and upper abdomen to show whole liver to exclude cardiorespiratory pathology.

Note

▦ Relevant clinical details are needed by the radiologist for correct radiological interpretation.

CASE STUDY 114: AP VIEW OF CHEST AND ABDOMEN OF PRETERM INFANT

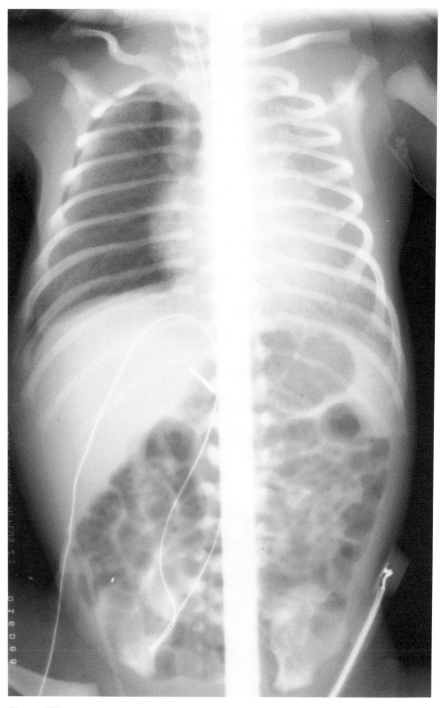

Figure 125

Technical comments

The infant has probably been removed only partly from the incubator so that the vertical perspex side of the incubator appears as a radio-opaque broad line along the length of the infant's spine. Exposure satisfactory (good detail seen in right lung); partial inspiratory film (8 posterior rib ends visible above right diaphragm); rotated to the right (asymmetry of rib cage and location of anterior rib ends); lordotic (upper ribs horizontal); head facing right.

Clinical equipment

A skin probe/sensor, left arm sphygmomanometer cuff, endotracheal tube (ETT) and umbilical arterial electrode (UAE) in situ.

Radiological interpretation

ETT tip at T2; UAE tip obscured by artefact. Artefact and rotation preclude interpretation of mediastinum and heart appearances. Small right pneumothorax. Liver on the right. Stomach and spleen on the left. Bowel gas shadows appear normal.

Conclusion

Technically unacceptable film which must be repeated. Small right pneumothorax in infant on intensive care.

CASE STUDY 115: AP VIEW OF CHEST AND ABDOMEN OF PRETERM INFANT

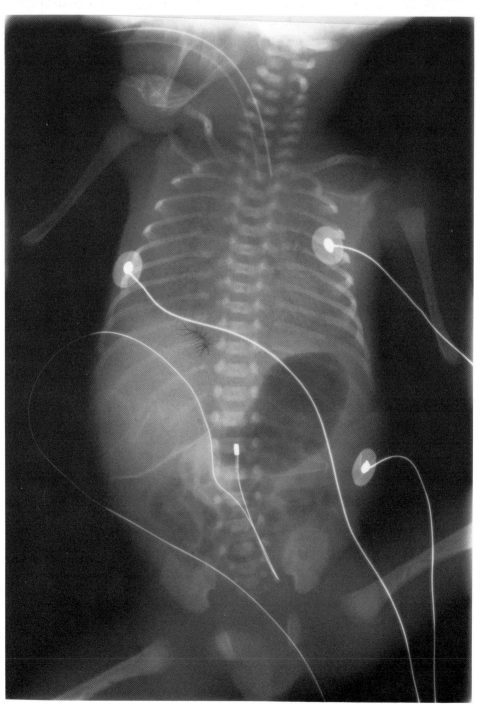

Figure 126

Technical comments

Slightly overexposed film; inspiratory film (9 posterior rib ends visible above right diaphragm); not rotated (anterior rib ends symmetrically placed); not lordotic (upper ribs appear to curve forwards and downwards); head facing right. Right chest ECG lead and UAC should have been removed from field of interest. Gonads irradiated.

Clinical equipment

Three ECG electrodes, endotracheal tube (ETT) and umbilical arterial catheter (UAC) electrode in situ.

Radiological interpretation

Mediastinum and heart appear normal. ETT tip at T2. Air in trachea and main bronchi clearly seen. Inadequate film for interpretation of lung field appearance. UAC electrode tip at T2. Diaphragms not clearly seen. Liver on the right. Stomach on the left. Bowel gas appearances normal. No gas in rectum. Black artefact over right upper abdomen is electrostatic. Multiple white line artefacts across abdomen are caused by dressings.

Conclusion

Technically inadequate film of chest and with multiple artefacts.

Suggest withdraw UAC electrode 1 cm and repeat chest and abdominal views separately.

Index